HEALING THROUGH FOOD

RECIPES FOR ANTI INFLAMMATORY AND AUTOIMMUNE DISEASES

OLIVIA WILSON

Copyright

TABLE OF CONTENTS

Chapter 1

Understanding the Anti-Inflammatory Diet

What is Inflammation?

- **Acute vs. chronic inflammation**

Inflammation is the body's natural defense mechanism, triggered when it encounters harmful stimuli such as infections, injuries, or toxins. However, the duration and nature of inflammation can have vastly different effects on your health.

1. Acute Inflammation

Definition:

A short-term, immediate response by the immune system to injury or infection. It aims to protect the body and promote healing.

Key Characteristics:

- Duration: Lasts from a few hours to a few days.

- Symptoms: Redness, swelling, heat, pain, and sometimes loss of function in the affected area.

- Purpose: Helps remove harmful agents (e.g., bacteria, damaged cells) and begins the healing process.

Examples of Acute Inflammation:

- A cut or scrape on the skin.

- Sore throat due to a viral or bacterial infection.

- Sprained ankle causing localized swelling and pain.

- Acute bronchitis or sinusitis.

Benefits:

- Protects the body from further damage.

- Initiates the repair process by increasing blood flow and immune cell activity.

Downside:

- If left unresolved or triggered too frequently, it may transition into chronic inflammation.

2. Chronic Inflammation

Definition:

A long-term, persistent inflammatory response that occurs even when there is no immediate injury or infection. It can damage healthy cells and tissues, contributing to the development of diseases.

Key Characteristics:

- Duration: Lasts for months or years.

- Symptoms: Often subtle and systemic, including fatigue, joint pain, digestive issues, and low-grade fever.

- Impact: Causes wear and tear on the body, potentially leading to chronic diseases.

Examples of Chronic Inflammation:

- Autoimmune diseases like rheumatoid arthritis, lupus, or Hashimoto's thyroiditis.

- Chronic conditions such as Type 2 diabetes, heart disease, or Alzheimer's.

- Long-term exposure to irritants (e.g., pollution, smoking, processed foods).

Causes:

- Persistent infections or injuries.

- Poor diet high in processed and inflammatory foods.

- Chronic stress, lack of sleep, and sedentary lifestyle.

- Genetic predisposition or immune system dysfunction.

Downside:

- Chronic inflammation is linked to a wide range of diseases, including cancer, cardiovascular disease, and neurodegenerative disorders.

- **Causes of chronic inflammation: stress, diet, lifestyle, environment**

Chronic inflammation occurs when the body's immune system remains active over a prolonged period, even in the absence of a direct threat. Various factors contribute to this persistent state of inflammation, including stress, poor diet, lifestyle choices, and environmental factors.

1. Stress

How Stress Triggers Inflammation:

- Chronic stress leads to an overproduction of cortisol, the stress hormone. Over time, the body becomes less sensitive to cortisol, which normally regulates inflammation.

- Prolonged stress also increases the production of pro-inflammatory cytokines, proteins that signal the immune system to remain active.

Examples of Stress-Related Triggers:

- Workplace pressure and deadlines.

- Family responsibilities or caregiving roles.

- Emotional trauma, anxiety, or depression.

Effects:

- Worsens existing conditions such as heart disease, autoimmune disorders, and digestive problems.

- Slows down the body's healing process.

2. Diet

How Diet Contributes to Chronic Inflammation:

- Pro-Inflammatory Foods: Diets high in processed, sugary, and fatty foods promote the production of inflammatory markers in the body.

- Gut Microbiome Imbalance: A poor diet disrupts the gut microbiota, causing a leaky gut, which allows toxins and bacteria to enter the bloodstream and trigger inflammation.

Pro-Inflammatory Foods to Avoid:

- Refined sugars and carbohydrates (e.g., soda, white bread).

- Trans fats (e.g., fried foods, margarine).

- Processed meats (e.g., bacon, hot dogs).

- Excessive alcohol and artificial additives.

Impact:

•	Poor nutrition not only promotes inflammation but also increases the risk of obesity, a major driver of inflammation.

3. Lifestyle Choices

Sedentary Lifestyle:

•	Lack of physical activity slows metabolism and increases fat accumulation, particularly visceral fat, which releases inflammatory substances called adipokines.

•	Prolonged sitting or inactivity contributes to stiffness, joint pain, and systemic inflammation.

Sleep Deprivation:

•	Poor sleep disrupts the circadian rhythm, leading to hormonal imbalances and increased levels of pro-inflammatory markers.

•	Chronic sleep loss can worsen inflammatory conditions such as arthritis and cardiovascular disease.

Smoking and Substance Use:

•	Smoking introduces toxins that directly damage cells and trigger an inflammatory response.

•	Excessive alcohol consumption damages the liver and intestines, leading to systemic inflammation.

4. Environmental Factors

Toxins and Pollutants:

•	Air pollution, pesticides, and chemicals found in cleaning products or plastics can trigger an immune response, leading to chronic inflammation.

- Heavy metals (e.g., lead, mercury) and industrial chemicals in the environment can accumulate in the body, overburdening the immune system.

Chronic Infections or Allergens:

- Persistent exposure to allergens, such as mold or pollen, keeps the immune system in an overactive state.

- Chronic infections (e.g., Epstein-Barr virus, Helicobacter pylori) can lead to low-grade, ongoing inflammation.

Urban Lifestyle:

- Noise pollution and exposure to constant artificial light (blue light from screens) disrupt sleep patterns and elevate stress hormones.

The Cycle of Chronic Inflammation

Many of these causes are interconnected:

- Stress can lead to poor sleep and unhealthy food choices.

- Environmental pollutants can worsen respiratory issues, leading to sedentary behavior.

- Poor lifestyle habits, in turn, worsen stress and inflammation, creating a vicious cycle.

Key Takeaway

By identifying and addressing these causes, you can reduce the body's inflammatory load and promote better health. The anti-inflammatory diet plays a crucial role in breaking this cycle by targeting key triggers, supporting the immune system, and restoring balance.

Why the Anti-Inflammatory Diet?

- **Reducing inflammation at the cellular level**

Understanding Cellular Inflammation

- Chronic inflammation starts at the cellular level when the immune system is triggered continuously. This can result in damaged tissues, oxidative stress, and the release of harmful inflammatory markers, such as cytokines and free radicals.

- Over time, this damage weakens cells, impairs their ability to repair themselves, and contributes to the progression of chronic diseases.

How Diet Plays a Role

- Antioxidant-Rich Foods: The anti-inflammatory diet emphasizes foods like berries, leafy greens, and nuts, which are rich in antioxidants. These substances neutralize free radicals, preventing cellular damage and reducing oxidative stress.

- Omega-3 Fatty Acids: Found in fatty fish, walnuts, and flaxseeds, omega-3s counteract pro-inflammatory omega-6 fatty acids, restoring balance and calming overactive immune responses.

- Phytonutrients: Compounds like flavonoids in fruits and vegetables protect cells by reducing inflammation and supporting detoxification.

Specific Benefits

1. Improved Cellular Repair: Nutrients like vitamin C (found in citrus fruits) and zinc (found in seeds and legumes) boost the body's ability to repair damaged cells.

2.   Reduced Chronic Disease Risk: By addressing inflammation at its source, the anti-inflammatory diet lowers the risk of conditions like arthritis, diabetes, heart disease, and neurodegenerative disorders.

3.   Enhanced Immune Function: A balanced immune response prevents the immune system from attacking healthy cells, which is particularly beneficial for autoimmune conditions.

4.   Balanced Hormones: Foods like turmeric, ginger, and leafy greens help modulate hormones like cortisol, reducing stress-induced inflammation.

The Power of Food as Medicine

The anti-inflammatory diet isn't a quick fix or fad—it's a lifestyle approach to healing. By focusing on nutrient-dense, whole foods, this diet provides your cells with the tools they need to thrive. Over time, consistent changes at the cellular level lead to improved energy, better digestion, enhanced mental clarity, and a reduced risk of chronic disease.

- **Its role in overall health and longevity**

The anti-inflammatory diet goes beyond managing chronic inflammation—it lays the foundation for a longer, healthier life. Chronic inflammation has been identified as a root cause of many age-related diseases, and addressing it through diet can enhance both the quality and length of life.

1. Preventing Age-Related Diseases

Chronic Diseases and Inflammation:

- Persistent, low-grade inflammation is a significant contributor to diseases like diabetes, heart disease, Alzheimer's, arthritis, and certain cancers.

- An anti-inflammatory diet reduces the production of pro-inflammatory markers, helping to prevent or manage these conditions.

14

Key Protective Foods:

- Fruits and Vegetables: High in vitamins, minerals, and antioxidants, these foods protect cells from damage caused by oxidative stress, a major driver of aging and inflammation.

- Healthy Fats: Omega-3 fatty acids (from fish, walnuts, and flaxseeds) and monounsaturated fats (from olive oil and avocados) promote heart health and reduce inflammation.

- Whole Grains and Legumes: These provide fiber, which supports gut health and helps regulate blood sugar levels, reducing inflammation and the risk of metabolic diseases.

2. Supporting Cellular Health

How Diet Influences Longevity:

- Reduced Oxidative Stress: The anti-inflammatory diet emphasizes antioxidant-rich foods, such as berries, green tea, and dark chocolate, which neutralize free radicals and protect cells.

- Enhanced Mitochondrial Function: Mitochondria, the "powerhouses" of cells, are particularly vulnerable to damage from inflammation. Nutrient-dense foods support their function, improving energy levels and slowing cellular aging.

- Telomere Protection: Telomeres, the protective caps on the ends of chromosomes, shorten with age and inflammation. Foods like nuts, seeds, and green vegetables have been linked to slower telomere shortening, which is associated with longer life expectancy.

3. Improving Mental and Emotional Well-being

Brain Health:

- Chronic inflammation is linked to cognitive decline, including Alzheimer's and other neurodegenerative diseases.

• Foods like turmeric (rich in curcumin), leafy greens, and fatty fish have anti-inflammatory properties that protect brain cells and improve memory and focus.

Mood Regulation:

• Inflammation in the brain has been associated with depression and anxiety.

• An anti-inflammatory diet, rich in omega-3s, magnesium, and B vitamins, supports neurotransmitter function and reduces inflammation, promoting emotional stability.

4. Promoting Gut Health

The Gut-Inflammation Connection:

• A significant portion of the immune system resides in the gut. Poor gut health can trigger systemic inflammation.

• The anti-inflammatory diet includes probiotics (yogurt, kefir, fermented vegetables) and prebiotics (garlic, onions, bananas) to balance gut bacteria, strengthen the gut lining, and reduce inflammation.

5. Extending Longevity

The Role of Inflammation in Aging:

• Chronic inflammation accelerates "inflammaging," a process where inflammation speeds up aging at the cellular level.

• By reducing inflammation, the anti-inflammatory diet helps slow down this process, improving overall vitality.

Longevity Hotspots:

• In regions like the Mediterranean and Okinawa, where people live longer, diets are naturally anti-inflammatory. These diets prioritize fresh vegetables, whole grains, nuts, healthy fats, and minimal processed foods.

Key Takeaway

An anti-inflammatory diet isn't just about managing symptoms; it's about optimizing your body's systems for long-term health and vitality. By reducing inflammation, you not only address current health issues but also set the stage for a longer, more vibrant life.

Diseases and Conditions it Can Help

*   **Autoimmune diseases (e.g., rheumatoid arthritis, lupus, Hashimoto's)**

Its Role in Overall Health and Longevity

The anti-inflammatory diet goes beyond managing chronic inflammation—it lays the foundation for a longer, healthier life. Chronic inflammation has been identified as a root cause of many age-related diseases, and addressing it through diet can enhance both the quality and length of life.

1. Preventing Age-Related Diseases

Chronic Diseases and Inflammation:

*   Persistent, low-grade inflammation is a significant contributor to diseases like diabetes, heart disease, Alzheimer's, arthritis, and certain cancers.

*   An anti-inflammatory diet reduces the production of pro-inflammatory markers, helping to prevent or manage these conditions.

Key Protective Foods:

- Fruits and Vegetables: High in vitamins, minerals, and antioxidants, these foods protect cells from damage caused by oxidative stress, a major driver of aging and inflammation.

- Healthy Fats: Omega-3 fatty acids (from fish, walnuts, and flaxseeds) and monounsaturated fats (from olive oil and avocados) promote heart health and reduce inflammation.

- Whole Grains and Legumes: These provide fiber, which supports gut health and helps regulate blood sugar levels, reducing inflammation and the risk of metabolic diseases.

2. Supporting Cellular Health

How Diet Influences Longevity:

- Reduced Oxidative Stress: The anti-inflammatory diet emphasizes antioxidant-rich foods, such as berries, green tea, and dark chocolate, which neutralize free radicals and protect cells.

- Enhanced Mitochondrial Function: Mitochondria, the "powerhouses" of cells, are particularly vulnerable to damage from inflammation. Nutrient-dense foods support their function, improving energy levels and slowing cellular aging.

- Telomere Protection: Telomeres, the protective caps on the ends of chromosomes, shorten with age and inflammation. Foods like nuts, seeds, and green vegetables have been linked to slower telomere shortening, which is associated with longer life expectancy.

3. Improving Mental and Emotional Well-being

Brain Health:

- Chronic inflammation is linked to cognitive decline, including Alzheimer's and other neurodegenerative diseases.

- Foods like turmeric (rich in curcumin), leafy greens, and fatty fish have anti-inflammatory properties that protect brain cells and improve memory and focus.

Mood Regulation:

- Inflammation in the brain has been associated with depression and anxiety.

- An anti-inflammatory diet, rich in omega-3s, magnesium, and B vitamins, supports neurotransmitter function and reduces inflammation, promoting emotional stability.

4. Promoting Gut Health

The Gut-Inflammation Connection:

- A significant portion of the immune system resides in the gut. Poor gut health can trigger systemic inflammation.

- The anti-inflammatory diet includes probiotics (yogurt, kefir, fermented vegetables) and prebiotics (garlic, onions, bananas) to balance gut bacteria, strengthen the gut lining, and reduce inflammation.

5. Extending Longevity

The Role of Inflammation in Aging:

- Chronic inflammation accelerates "inflammaging," a process where inflammation speeds up aging at the cellular level.

- By reducing inflammation, the anti-inflammatory diet helps slow down this process, improving overall vitality.

Longevity Hotspots:

- In regions like the Mediterranean and Okinawa, where people live longer, diets are naturally anti-inflammatory. These diets prioritize fresh vegetables, whole grains, nuts, healthy fats, and minimal processed foods.

> • **Chronic diseases (e.g., heart disease, diabetes, cancer, Alzheimer's)**

Chronic diseases such as heart disease, diabetes, cancer, and Alzheimer's are among the leading causes of death worldwide. A growing body of research links these conditions to persistent, low-grade inflammation in the body. Understanding how chronic inflammation contributes to these diseases—and how dietary changes can mitigate it—offers a powerful approach to prevention and management.

1. Heart Disease

Inflammation's Role:

• Chronic inflammation damages the lining of blood vessels, leading to the buildup of plaque (atherosclerosis).

• This increases the risk of heart attack, stroke, and hypertension.

Key Factors:

• High levels of inflammatory markers like C-reactive protein (CRP) are often found in individuals with heart disease.

• Diets high in trans fats, refined sugars, and processed foods exacerbate inflammation and contribute to plaque formation.

How the Anti-Inflammatory Diet Helps:

• Omega-3 Fatty Acids: Found in fatty fish, flaxseeds, and walnuts, these fats reduce inflammation and improve heart health.

• Antioxidant-Rich Foods: Leafy greens, berries, and nuts protect blood vessels from oxidative damage.

• Whole Grains: High in fiber, these help lower cholesterol levels and reduce inflammation.

2. Type 2 Diabetes

Inflammation's Role:

• Chronic inflammation impairs the body's ability to regulate blood sugar, contributing to insulin resistance.

• Visceral fat, often linked to obesity, produces pro-inflammatory substances that exacerbate the condition.

Key Factors:

• High levels of inflammatory cytokines disrupt insulin signaling pathways.

• A diet high in refined carbohydrates and sugars worsens blood sugar control and inflammation.

How the Anti-Inflammatory Diet Helps:

• Low-Glycemic Foods: Foods like sweet potatoes, quinoa, and legumes help stabilize blood sugar.

• Healthy Fats: Avocados, nuts, and seeds support insulin sensitivity and reduce inflammation.

• Spices: Turmeric and cinnamon have been shown to improve blood sugar regulation and combat inflammation.

3. Cancer

Inflammation's Role:

• Chronic inflammation creates an environment that encourages the growth and spread of cancer cells.

• Persistent immune activity can damage DNA and promote mutations that lead to cancer.

Key Factors:

- Inflammatory markers like COX-2 enzymes and cytokines contribute to tumor development.

- Obesity and diets high in processed foods, red meat, and alcohol are linked to increased cancer risk.

How the Anti-Inflammatory Diet Helps:

- Cruciferous Vegetables: Broccoli, cauliflower, and Brussels sprouts contain compounds that inhibit cancer cell growth.

- Brightly Colored Fruits: Blueberries, oranges, and cherries are rich in antioxidants that protect cells from DNA damage.

- Green Tea: Contains catechins, which reduce oxidative stress and inflammation associated with cancer.

4. Alzheimer's Disease

Inflammation's Role:

- Chronic inflammation in the brain contributes to the buildup of beta-amyloid plaques, a hallmark of Alzheimer's disease.

- Overactive immune responses in the brain (neuroinflammation) accelerate cognitive decline.

Key Factors:

- Elevated levels of inflammatory markers like interleukin-6 (IL-6) and tumor necrosis factor-alpha (TNF-α) are often seen in individuals with Alzheimer's.

- Diets high in refined sugars and unhealthy fats increase oxidative stress and neuroinflammation.

How the Anti-Inflammatory Diet Helps:

- Fatty Fish: Rich in DHA, an omega-3 fatty acid crucial for brain health.

•   Leafy Greens: Spinach, kale, and collards provide folate and vitamin K, which protect brain cells.

•   Spices: Curcumin in turmeric crosses the blood-brain barrier to reduce neuroinflammation and improve memory.

The Common Thread: Chronic Inflammation

While these diseases vary in their specific mechanisms, they all share a common link: chronic inflammation. This makes addressing inflammation a powerful strategy for preventing and managing these conditions.

Key Takeaway

An anti-inflammatory diet not only reduces inflammation but also addresses risk factors associated with chronic diseases. By nourishing the body with the right nutrients, it is possible to promote healing, prevent disease progression, and enhance overall health.

Would you like me to include additional details on specific foods, lifestyle changes, or scientific studies supporting these claims?

•   **Skin conditions (e.g., psoriasis, eczema)**

Chronic inflammation plays a significant role in many skin conditions, including psoriasis and eczema. These conditions arise from an overactive immune response, leading to redness, itching, flaking, and other skin-related symptoms. An anti-inflammatory diet can help manage these symptoms by addressing inflammation at its root and providing the skin with the nutrients it needs to heal.

1. Psoriasis

Inflammation's Role:

- Psoriasis is an autoimmune condition where the immune system mistakenly attacks healthy skin cells, causing an overproduction of skin cells.

- This results in thick, scaly patches of skin, often accompanied by redness and irritation.

Key Factors:

- Inflammatory markers like interleukin-17 (IL-17) and tumor necrosis factor-alpha (TNF-α) are elevated in individuals with psoriasis.

- Triggers such as stress, diet, infections, and environmental factors can exacerbate symptoms.

How the Anti-Inflammatory Diet Helps:

- Fatty Fish: Rich in omega-3 fatty acids, salmon and mackerel reduce skin inflammation and improve symptoms.

- Colorful Vegetables: Carrots, sweet potatoes, and bell peppers provide beta-carotene and vitamin A, which promote skin health.

- Spices: Turmeric and ginger help suppress inflammatory pathways linked to psoriasis flare-ups.

2. Eczema

Inflammation's Role:

- Eczema, or atopic dermatitis, is characterized by itchy, inflamed, and dry skin caused by an overactive immune response and a weakened skin barrier.

- Chronic inflammation disrupts the skin's ability to retain moisture and defend against irritants.

Key Factors:

• Triggers include allergens, environmental irritants, stress, and diet.

• Imbalances in gut health, such as dysbiosis (an imbalance of gut bacteria), can contribute to inflammation and worsen eczema symptoms.

How the Anti-Inflammatory Diet Helps:

• Probiotic-Rich Foods: Yogurt, kefir, and fermented vegetables improve gut health and strengthen the skin barrier.

• Healthy Fats: Avocados, nuts, and seeds provide essential fatty acids that keep skin hydrated and reduce irritation.

• Vitamin C-Rich Foods: Oranges, strawberries, and kale support collagen production and help repair damaged skin.

3. The Gut-Skin Connection

• A healthy gut is essential for healthy skin. Imbalances in the gut microbiome can trigger systemic inflammation, leading to skin conditions like eczema and psoriasis.

• An anti-inflammatory diet that includes prebiotics (garlic, onions, bananas) and probiotics supports gut health, reducing inflammation and improving skin symptoms.

4. Supporting Skin Healing with Nutrients

• Zinc: Found in pumpkin seeds and lentils, zinc supports skin repair and reduces inflammation.

• Vitamin E: Present in almonds, sunflower seeds, and spinach, vitamin E protects the skin from oxidative damage.

• Polyphenols: Compounds in green tea and dark chocolate have anti-inflammatory properties that benefit the skin.

Key Takeaway

Skin conditions like psoriasis and eczema are deeply connected to inflammation. By adopting an anti-inflammatory diet rich in omega-3s, antioxidants, probiotics, and essential nutrients, it is possible to calm the immune system, reduce flare-ups, and promote healthier skin.

- **Digestive disorders (e.g., Crohn's, IBS, leaky gut syndrome)**

Digestive disorders like Crohn's disease, irritable bowel syndrome (IBS), and leaky gut syndrome are closely linked to chronic inflammation in the gastrointestinal (GI) tract. This inflammation disrupts digestion, impairs nutrient absorption, and can lead to systemic health issues. An anti-inflammatory diet helps restore balance in the gut, support the intestinal lining, and reduce inflammation, making it a cornerstone of managing these conditions.

1. Crohn's Disease

Inflammation's Role:

- Crohn's is a chronic inflammatory bowel disease (IBD) that causes inflammation in any part of the GI tract, often leading to abdominal pain, diarrhea, weight loss, and malnutrition.

- Persistent inflammation can damage the intestinal lining, resulting in ulcers and scar tissue.

Key Factors:

- Triggers include a dysregulated immune response, gut bacteria imbalances, and dietary irritants like processed foods and high-sugar diets.

How the Anti-Inflammatory Diet Helps:

- Easily Digestible Proteins: Bone broth, lean poultry, and fish provide essential amino acids that aid tissue repair.

- Omega-3 Fatty Acids: Found in salmon, chia seeds, and flaxseeds, they reduce intestinal inflammation.

- Low-FODMAP Foods: These are less likely to ferment in the gut and reduce symptoms of bloating and diarrhea during flares.

2. Irritable Bowel Syndrome (IBS)

Inflammation's Role:

- IBS involves abdominal discomfort, bloating, gas, and irregular bowel movements. While it's not classified as inflammatory, chronic low-grade inflammation often exacerbates symptoms.

- Stress, food sensitivities, and gut dysbiosis are common triggers.

Key Factors:

- IBS is often associated with a disrupted gut-brain axis and altered gut microbiota.

- Foods like gluten, dairy, and artificial sweeteners may worsen symptoms.

How the Anti-Inflammatory Diet Helps:

- Probiotic-Rich Foods: Fermented foods like sauerkraut and kimchi help balance gut bacteria and alleviate symptoms.

- High-Fiber Foods: Soluble fiber from oats, bananas, and sweet potatoes soothes the digestive tract and regulates bowel movements.

- Herbs and Spices: Ginger and peppermint reduce bloating and cramping by relaxing the intestinal muscles.

3. Leaky Gut Syndrome

Inflammation's Role:

- In leaky gut syndrome, the intestinal lining becomes permeable, allowing undigested food particles, toxins, and pathogens to "leak" into the bloodstream.

- This triggers an immune response and systemic inflammation, often linked to autoimmune diseases, allergies, and chronic fatigue.

Key Factors:

- Causes include poor diet (high in processed foods and sugar), stress, infections, and imbalanced gut bacteria.

- Inflammatory foods like gluten, alcohol, and fried foods worsen gut permeability.

How the Anti-Inflammatory Diet Helps:

- Collagen-Rich Foods: Bone broth and collagen peptides support the repair of the intestinal lining.

- Gut-Healing Nutrients: Zinc (found in pumpkin seeds) and glutamine (in spinach and cabbage) help rebuild the gut barrier.

- Anti-Inflammatory Foods: Turmeric, leafy greens, and berries combat inflammation and oxidative stress in the gut.

The Gut-Inflammation Connection

All these conditions highlight the importance of maintaining a healthy gut environment. Chronic inflammation disrupts the microbiome and intestinal lining, leading to a cycle of poor digestion, nutrient deficiencies, and worsening inflammation.

4. Foods to Prioritize

- Probiotics: Yogurt, kefir, miso, and tempeh to support a healthy microbiome.

- Prebiotics: Garlic, onions, asparagus, and bananas to feed beneficial gut bacteria.

- Omega-3s: Salmon, chia seeds, and walnuts to reduce intestinal inflammation.

- Low-Glycemic Foods: Whole grains, lentils, and vegetables to stabilize blood sugar and reduce inflammatory spikes.

5. Foods to Avoid

- Processed foods high in sugar, trans fats, and artificial additives.

- Gluten and dairy (if sensitivities exist).

- Alcohol, caffeine, and spicy foods that irritate the gut lining.

Key Takeaway

Digestive disorders are deeply connected to inflammation, making an anti-inflammatory diet essential for healing. By focusing on nutrient-dense, gut-friendly foods and avoiding irritants, it's possible to reduce inflammation, improve digestion, and support overall gut health.

How It Works

- **Eliminating pro-inflammatory foods (e.g., refined sugar, trans fats)**

Chronic inflammation often stems from dietary habits, with certain foods acting as major contributors to inflammation in the body. By eliminating these pro-inflammatory foods, we can reduce the strain on the immune system, improve cellular health, and support overall well-being.

1. Refined Sugar

Why It's Inflammatory:

•   Consuming excess refined sugar spikes blood sugar levels, causing the body to release insulin and pro-inflammatory cytokines.

•   Over time, these spikes can lead to insulin resistance, oxidative stress, and chronic inflammation.

Where It's Found:

•   Sweets, baked goods, sugary beverages, and processed foods.

•   Hidden sources include sauces (ketchup, barbecue sauce) and flavored yogurts.

Better Alternatives:

•   Natural sweeteners like honey, maple syrup (in moderation), or stevia.

•   Use whole fruits to add natural sweetness.

2. Trans Fats

Why They're Inflammatory:

•   Trans fats (partially hydrogenated oils) disrupt the balance between good and bad cholesterol, increasing LDL (bad cholesterol) and decreasing HDL (good cholesterol).

•   They contribute to systemic inflammation, increasing the risk of heart disease and other chronic conditions.

Where They're Found:

•   Processed and packaged snacks (chips, cookies).

•   Margarine, shortening, and fried fast foods.

Better Alternatives:

• Use healthy fats like olive oil, avocado oil, or coconut oil for cooking.

• Snack on nuts, seeds, and whole-grain options instead of processed foods.

3. Refined Carbohydrates

Why They're Inflammatory:

• Refined carbs like white bread, white rice, and pastries are quickly broken down into glucose, causing rapid blood sugar spikes.

• High glycemic index foods promote insulin resistance and inflammation.

Where They're Found:

• White bread, white pasta, instant rice, and most breakfast cereals.

Better Alternatives:

• Whole grains such as quinoa, brown rice, oats, and whole-grain bread.

• Legumes like lentils, chickpeas, and black beans provide slow-digesting carbohydrates.

4. Processed Meats

Why They're Inflammatory:

• Processed meats are high in advanced glycation end products (AGEs) and saturated fats, which promote inflammation.

• They've been linked to an increased risk of heart disease, cancer, and other inflammatory conditions.

Where They're Found:

- Bacon, sausage, hot dogs, deli meats, and smoked meats.

Better Alternatives:

- Opt for lean, unprocessed proteins like chicken, turkey, fish, or plant-based options like tofu and tempeh.

5. Artificial Additives and Preservatives

Why They're Inflammatory:

- Artificial sweeteners (e.g., aspartame) and preservatives (e.g., sulfites, nitrates) can disrupt the gut microbiome and trigger immune responses.

- Over time, these substances contribute to systemic inflammation and oxidative stress.

Where They're Found:

- Diet sodas, sugar-free snacks, packaged foods, and fast food.

Better Alternatives:

- Choose whole, minimally processed foods.

- Read labels and avoid foods with long lists of unrecognizable ingredients.

6. Alcohol

Why It's Inflammatory:

- Excessive alcohol consumption damages the liver, disrupts gut health, and increases inflammatory markers.

- Chronic alcohol use is associated with conditions like leaky gut syndrome and liver inflammation.

Where It's Found:

•	Beer, wine, and spirits.

Better Alternatives:

•	Drink alcohol in moderation (if at all), choosing options like red wine, which contains anti-inflammatory polyphenols.

•	Substitute with herbal teas, sparkling water, or mocktails using fresh fruits and herbs.

•	**Emphasizing anti-inflammatory nutrients (e.g., omega-3s, antioxidants, polyphenols)**

An anti-inflammatory diet is built around foods rich in specific nutrients that naturally combat inflammation. These nutrients work at the cellular level to protect against oxidative stress, repair tissue damage, and regulate immune responses. By incorporating foods high in omega-3 fatty acids, antioxidants, and polyphenols, you can support the body's natural defenses and promote overall health.

1. Omega-3 Fatty Acids

Why They're Anti-Inflammatory:

•	Omega-3s reduce the production of pro-inflammatory molecules and cytokines.

•	They support heart, brain, and joint health, making them essential for managing chronic inflammatory conditions.

Sources:

•	Fatty Fish: Salmon, mackerel, sardines, herring, and tuna.

•	Plant-Based Options: Chia seeds, flaxseeds, walnuts, and hemp seeds.

- Supplements: High-quality fish oil or algae-based omega-3 supplements.

How to Incorporate:

- Add chia seeds or ground flaxseeds to smoothies or oatmeal.

- Grill or bake salmon for a flavorful, nutrient-rich dinner.

2. Antioxidants

Why They're Anti-Inflammatory:

- Antioxidants neutralize free radicals, which cause oxidative stress and inflammation.

- They protect cells from damage, reduce aging-related inflammation, and support immune health.

Sources:

- Fruits: Berries (blueberries, strawberries, raspberries), oranges, and pomegranates.

- Vegetables: Kale, spinach, sweet potatoes, and bell peppers.

- Other Foods: Dark chocolate (70% or higher cacao) and green tea.

How to Incorporate:

- Snack on a mixed berry fruit bowl or top yogurt with fresh berries.

- Blend leafy greens like kale or spinach into a smoothie.

3. Polyphenols

Why They're Anti-Inflammatory:

- Polyphenols are plant compounds that reduce inflammation by modulating gut bacteria, improving cell signaling, and reducing oxidative stress.

- They've been linked to reduced risks of heart disease, diabetes, and neurodegenerative diseases.

Sources:

- Herbs and Spices: Turmeric (curcumin), ginger, garlic, and cinnamon.

- Beverages: Green tea, black tea, and coffee (in moderation).

- Other Foods: Olives, extra virgin olive oil, dark chocolate, and grapes.

How to Incorporate:

- Use turmeric and ginger in soups, curries, or teas.

- Drizzle olive oil over salads or roasted vegetables.

4. Fiber

Why It's Anti-Inflammatory:

- Fiber feeds beneficial gut bacteria, which produce anti-inflammatory compounds like short-chain fatty acids.

- It regulates blood sugar and reduces inflammation associated with insulin resistance.

Sources:

- Whole grains (quinoa, oats, barley), legumes (lentils, chickpeas), fruits, and vegetables.

How to Incorporate:

- Make hearty grain bowls with quinoa and roasted vegetables.

- Add legumes to soups, stews, or salads.

5. Vitamin D

Why It's Anti-Inflammatory:

- Vitamin D modulates the immune system and helps reduce chronic inflammation.

- Low vitamin D levels are associated with autoimmune diseases and increased inflammation.

Sources:

- Fatty fish (salmon, tuna, sardines), egg yolks, fortified foods (milk, cereals), and sunlight exposure.

How to Incorporate:

- Include fatty fish in your weekly meals.

- Consider a supplement if natural intake is insufficient, especially during winter months.

6. Probiotics and Prebiotics

Why They're Anti-Inflammatory:

- Probiotics improve gut health by balancing the microbiome, which plays a critical role in inflammation regulation.

- Prebiotics feed beneficial bacteria, enhancing their anti-inflammatory effects.

Sources:

- Probiotics: Yogurt, kefir, sauerkraut, kimchi, and miso.

- Prebiotics: Garlic, onions, asparagus, bananas, and oats.

How to Incorporate:

- Include a serving of fermented foods daily.

- Add prebiotic-rich vegetables to stir-fries, soups, or salads.

- **Restoring gut health and reducing oxidative stress**

Your gut and cellular health are deeply connected to inflammation in the body. An imbalanced gut microbiome and excessive oxidative stress can contribute to chronic inflammation, affecting everything from digestion to immune function. By focusing on gut health and minimizing oxidative stress, you can restore balance and enhance your body's ability to fight inflammation naturally.

Why Gut Health Matters

- The gut microbiome, home to trillions of bacteria, plays a critical role in digestion, immunity, and inflammation regulation.

- An unhealthy gut, often caused by poor diet, stress, or medications, can lead to "leaky gut" syndrome, where toxins and undigested food particles enter the bloodstream, triggering inflammation.

Steps to Restore Gut Health

1. Consume Probiotic-Rich Foods

Probiotics replenish beneficial bacteria in the gut, improving digestion and reducing inflammation.

- Sources: Yogurt (unsweetened), kefir, sauerkraut, kimchi, miso, and tempeh.

2. Incorporate Prebiotic-Rich Foods

Prebiotics feed the beneficial bacteria, helping them thrive and maintain balance.

•   Sources: Garlic, onions, asparagus, bananas, apples, and whole grains.

3.   Eat Fiber-Rich Foods

Fiber supports gut bacteria and promotes the production of anti-inflammatory short-chain fatty acids.

•   Sources: Legumes, vegetables, fruits, nuts, and seeds.

4.   Avoid Gut Irritants

Eliminate or reduce foods that disrupt gut health, such as:

•   Refined sugar, alcohol, artificial sweeteners, and heavily processed foods.

5.   Stay Hydrated

Proper hydration supports digestion and the elimination of waste products that can irritate the gut lining.

6.   Manage Stress

Chronic stress can disrupt the gut-brain connection, leading to inflammation and digestive issues.

•   Practice mindfulness, yoga, deep breathing, or other relaxation techniques to support gut health.

Reducing Oxidative Stress

What Is Oxidative Stress?

•   Oxidative stress occurs when there is an imbalance between free radicals (unstable molecules) and antioxidants in the body.

- Excessive oxidative stress damages cells, proteins, and DNA, leading to chronic inflammation and diseases like heart disease, cancer, and diabetes.

Steps to Reduce Oxidative Stress

1. Increase Antioxidant Intake

Antioxidants neutralize free radicals, preventing cellular damage.

- Sources:

- Fruits: Berries, citrus fruits, grapes, and cherries.

- Vegetables: Spinach, kale, broccoli, and sweet potatoes.

- Others: Green tea, dark chocolate, and nuts (e.g., walnuts, almonds).

2. Incorporate Anti-Inflammatory Spices

Spices like turmeric (curcumin) and ginger have potent antioxidant and anti-inflammatory properties.

- How to Use: Add to teas, soups, smoothies, or roasted vegetables.

3. Choose Healthy Fats

Omega-3 fatty acids and monounsaturated fats help reduce oxidative stress and inflammation.

- Sources: Fatty fish, flaxseeds, chia seeds, olive oil, and avocados.

4. Limit Exposure to Toxins

Reduce contact with environmental toxins that contribute to free radical formation, such as:

- Smoking, pollution, and pesticides.

5. Exercise Regularly

Moderate exercise boosts antioxidant defenses while reducing inflammation.

- Avoid overtraining, which can increase oxidative stress.

6. Get Enough Sleep

Poor sleep disrupts the body's ability to repair oxidative damage. Aim for 7–9 hours of quality sleep each night.

Key Synergy Between Gut Health and Oxidative Stress

- A healthy gut enhances nutrient absorption, including antioxidants, which protect against oxidative stress.

- Similarly, reducing oxidative stress supports gut lining integrity and the microbiome, creating a positive feedback loop for reducing inflammation.

By focusing on gut health and combating oxidative stress, you can address two root causes of inflammation, paving the way for improved overall health.

The Science Behind It

- **Studies linking diet to inflammation**

Research consistently demonstrates the connection between diet and inflammation. Certain foods can either trigger or mitigate inflammatory responses in the body, significantly influencing chronic disease development and overall health. Below are key findings from studies that highlight the relationship between diet and inflammation:

1. The Role of Pro-Inflammatory Foods

Refined Sugar and Processed Foods

A study published in the Journal of Clinical Investigation (2017) found that diets high in refined sugar and processed foods contribute to increased levels of inflammatory markers, such as C-reactive protein (CRP). Excess sugar triggers the production of cytokines, which are signaling molecules that promote inflammation.

- Key Insight: Diets rich in processed foods and sugary beverages are linked to higher risks of heart disease, diabetes, and obesity.

Trans Fats and Inflammation

A 2019 meta-analysis in Nutrients reviewed the impact of trans fats on inflammation. Researchers observed that trans fats, found in fried foods, margarine, and baked goods, elevate CRP and interleukin-6 (IL-6) levels, both of which are markers of chronic inflammation.

- Key Insight: Eliminating trans fats can significantly reduce inflammation and improve cardiovascular health.

2. The Benefits of Anti-Inflammatory Diets

Mediterranean Diet

The Mediterranean diet is one of the most researched anti-inflammatory eating patterns. A 2018 study in The Lancet demonstrated that this diet—rich in fruits, vegetables, olive oil, nuts, and fatty fish—reduces inflammation and lowers the risk of cardiovascular disease, diabetes, and neurodegenerative disorders.

- Key Finding: Participants who followed the Mediterranean diet had lower levels of CRP and other inflammatory biomarkers compared to those on a Western diet.

Omega-3 Fatty Acids and Inflammation

A 2020 study in Frontiers in Nutrition highlighted the role of omega-3 fatty acids in reducing inflammation. Omega-3s, found in fatty fish and seeds, inhibit the production of pro-inflammatory molecules like prostaglandins and leukotrienes.

- Key Insight: Regular consumption of omega-3s is associated with reduced symptoms of arthritis, asthma, and other inflammatory conditions.

3. Gut Health and Inflammation

Fiber and Short-Chain Fatty Acids (SCFAs)

Research in Cell Host & Microbe (2019) explored the connection between dietary fiber, gut health, and inflammation. High-fiber diets promote the growth of beneficial gut bacteria that produce SCFAs, which have powerful anti-inflammatory effects.

- Key Insight: Low fiber intake leads to gut dysbiosis, increasing systemic inflammation and the risk of diseases like Crohn's and IBS.

Probiotics and Prebiotics

A systematic review in Nutrients (2021) found that probiotics (e.g., yogurt, kefir) and prebiotics (e.g., garlic, onions) restore gut microbiota balance and reduce inflammation markers.

- Key Insight: Gut health is closely tied to systemic inflammation and immune function.

4. Plant-Based Diets and Inflammation

Studies have consistently shown that plant-based diets reduce inflammation by providing abundant antioxidants, polyphenols, and fiber. A 2022 study in Advances in Nutrition found that participants following a plant-based diet had significantly lower levels of CRP and other inflammatory markers than those on an omnivorous diet.

•	Key Finding: A diet centered on whole grains, fruits, vegetables, nuts, and seeds is protective against inflammatory-related chronic diseases.

5. Effects of High Glycemic Index (GI) Foods

High-GI foods, like white bread and sugary snacks, cause rapid spikes in blood sugar levels, triggering an inflammatory response. A 2020 study in the American Journal of Clinical Nutrition demonstrated that diets high in high-GI foods lead to elevated levels of CRP and tumor necrosis factor-alpha (TNF-α).

•	Key Insight: Replacing high-GI foods with whole grains and low-GI alternatives reduces inflammation and stabilizes blood sugar.

6. Emerging Research on Spices and Herbs

Turmeric (Curcumin)

A 2021 meta-analysis in Critical Reviews in Food Science and Nutrition confirmed that curcumin, the active compound in turmeric, significantly reduces inflammatory markers like CRP and IL-6.

•	Key Insight: Curcumin has therapeutic potential for managing arthritis, metabolic syndrome, and other inflammatory conditions.

Ginger and Garlic

Studies published in Phytotherapy Research (2022) show that ginger and garlic have potent anti-inflammatory and antioxidant properties, reducing pain and inflammation in conditions like osteoarthritis.

Key Takeaways from Research

•	Diet plays a critical role in regulating inflammation. Foods rich in antioxidants, omega-3s, and fiber are consistently linked to reduced inflammatory markers.

• Avoiding pro-inflammatory foods like refined sugars, trans fats, and processed products can significantly lower chronic inflammation levels.

• Emerging research highlights the potential of specific dietary patterns, such as the Mediterranean or plant-based diets, to combat inflammation and promote overall health.

• **Role of plant-based foods, herbs, and spices**

A predominantly plant-based diet, complemented by anti-inflammatory herbs and spices, provides essential nutrients and bioactive compounds that combat chronic inflammation at its root. From antioxidants to phytonutrients, these foods not only reduce inflammation but also support overall health and disease prevention.

How Plant-Based Foods Fight Inflammation

Rich in Antioxidants

Plant-based foods are packed with antioxidants like vitamins C and E, beta-carotene, and flavonoids, which neutralize free radicals that contribute to oxidative stress and inflammation.

• Example: Berries, such as blueberries and raspberries, are high in anthocyanins, which have been shown to reduce inflammation and oxidative stress.

Loaded with Fiber

Fiber, abundant in plant-based foods, feeds beneficial gut bacteria that produce short-chain fatty acids (SCFAs). These SCFAs have potent anti-inflammatory effects.

• Example: Whole grains, legumes, and vegetables are excellent sources of dietary fiber that promote gut health and lower systemic inflammation.

Source of Polyphenols

Polyphenols are plant compounds with powerful anti-inflammatory and antioxidant properties.

• Example: Dark leafy greens (e.g., spinach, kale) and fruits like apples and grapes contain polyphenols that reduce inflammation and protect against chronic diseases.

Omega-3 Fatty Acids

While plant-based diets are often low in omega-6 fatty acids (pro-inflammatory when consumed in excess), they can be rich in omega-3s if specific foods are included.

• Example: Flaxseeds, chia seeds, and walnuts are plant-based sources of omega-3s that lower inflammation.

The Role of Herbs and Spices in Combating Inflammation

Turmeric (Curcumin)

• Active Compound: Curcumin, a potent anti-inflammatory and antioxidant.

• Benefits: Reduces markers of inflammation like CRP and helps manage chronic conditions like arthritis and metabolic syndrome.

• How to Use: Add turmeric to curries, teas, or golden milk for a daily anti-inflammatory boost.

Ginger

• Active Compounds: Gingerols and shogaols, which inhibit inflammatory pathways.

• Benefits: Reduces muscle pain, joint stiffness, and symptoms of digestive inflammation (e.g., IBS).

• How to Use: Use fresh or powdered ginger in teas, soups, or smoothies.

Garlic

• Active Compound: Allicin, known for its anti-inflammatory and antimicrobial properties.

• Benefits: Lowers CRP levels and supports immune function, particularly in heart health.

• How to Use: Incorporate raw or cooked garlic into savory dishes.

Cinnamon

• Active Compounds: Cinnamaldehyde and other polyphenols.

• Benefits: Reduces inflammation, balances blood sugar levels, and combats oxidative stress.

• How to Use: Sprinkle cinnamon on oatmeal, yogurt, or baked goods.

Rosemary

• Active Compounds: Rosmarinic acid and carnosol.

• Benefits: Reduces inflammation in joints and supports brain health by combating neuroinflammation.

• How to Use: Add rosemary to roasted vegetables, soups, or marinades.

Basil

• Active Compound: Eugenol, a natural anti-inflammatory agent.

• Benefits: Helps reduce swelling and inflammation in arthritis and other inflammatory conditions.

- How to Use: Use fresh basil in salads, pestos, or sauces.

Cloves

- Active Compounds: Eugenol and flavonoids.

- Benefits: Powerful antioxidant properties help combat inflammation and pain.

- How to Use: Add cloves to teas, curries, or baked dishes.

Incorporating Plant-Based Foods, Herbs, and Spices

Daily Checklist for Anti-Inflammatory Nutrition

1. Fruits and Vegetables: Aim for a variety of colors to maximize antioxidants and phytonutrients.

- Examples: Sweet potatoes, bell peppers, broccoli, and citrus fruits.

2. Whole Grains and Legumes: Choose complex carbohydrates that provide fiber and reduce inflammation.

- Examples: Quinoa, lentils, and chickpeas.

3. Nuts and Seeds: Include a handful of nuts or seeds daily for healthy fats and anti-inflammatory compounds.

- Examples: Almonds, sunflower seeds, and flaxseeds.

4. Herbs and Spices: Use fresh or dried herbs and spices liberally in cooking for flavor and health benefits.

Research Highlights

1. Turmeric and Curcumin

- A 2021 meta-analysis published in Critical Reviews in Food Science and Nutrition found that curcumin significantly reduces inflammatory biomarkers like CRP and IL-6, making it effective for managing chronic inflammation.z

2. Plant-Based Diets

• A 2022 study in Advances in Nutrition showed that plant-based diets lower CRP levels and protect against inflammatory-related diseases such as heart disease and diabetes.

3. Garlic and Ginger

• Studies in Phytotherapy Research (2020) demonstrated that garlic and ginger reduce oxidative stress and inflammation, particularly in conditions like arthritis and metabolic syndrome.

By emphasizing plant-based foods, herbs, and spices, you can create a diet that naturally reduces inflammation while providing essential nutrients for overall health. Would you like to expand this section with specific recipes that showcase these ingredients?

Chapter 2

Energizing Breakfasts (10 Recipes)

1. Golden Turmeric Overnight Oats

This vibrant and anti-inflammatory breakfast is packed with fiber, antioxidants, and the powerful properties of turmeric. Perfect for busy mornings, this recipe is quick, easy, and satisfying.

Ingredients (Serves 1)

- 1/2 cup rolled oats (gluten-free if needed)

- 1/2 cup unsweetened almond milk (or any milk of choice)

- 1/4 cup plain Greek yogurt (optional for added creaminess and protein)

- 1/2 tsp ground turmeric

- 1/4 tsp ground cinnamon

- 1/4 tsp ground ginger

- 1 tsp honey or maple syrup (optional, for sweetness)

- 1 tbsp chia seeds

- 1/2 tsp vanilla extract

- Pinch of black pepper (to enhance turmeric absorption)

- Optional toppings: Fresh berries, sliced banana, chopped nuts, shredded coconut

Instructions

1.   Mix Ingredients: In a jar or bowl, combine the oats, almond milk, yogurt (if using), turmeric, cinnamon, ginger, chia seeds, vanilla extract, black pepper, and sweetener (if desired). Stir well to combine.

2.   Refrigerate: Cover and refrigerate overnight (or at least 4-6 hours) to allow the oats to absorb the liquid and soften.

3.   Add Toppings: In the morning, give the oats a good stir and adjust the consistency with a splash of milk if needed. Add your favorite toppings like fresh berries, banana slices, or nuts.

4.   Serve and Enjoy: Enjoy your golden turmeric oats cold or warm them up in the microwave for 30-60 seconds if preferred.

Why It's Anti-Inflammatory

•   Turmeric: Contains curcumin, a potent anti-inflammatory compound.

•   Cinnamon and Ginger: Both are known for their ability to reduce inflammation and improve digestion.

•   Chia Seeds: High in omega-3 fatty acids and fiber, which support gut health and reduce systemic inflammation.

•   Berries and Nuts (Toppings): Rich in antioxidants and healthy fats to combat oxidative stress.

2.   Sweet Potato and Kale Breakfast Hash

This hearty and nutrient-dense breakfast is loaded with anti-inflammatory ingredients like sweet potatoes, kale, and spices. It's a perfect way to fuel your morning with vitamins, fiber, and healthy fats.

Ingredients (Serves 2)

- 1 large sweet potato, peeled and diced into small cubes

- 2 tbsp olive oil or avocado oil

- 1 small red onion, diced

- 1 red bell pepper, diced

- 2 cups fresh kale, stems removed and leaves chopped

- 2 garlic cloves, minced

- 1/2 tsp ground turmeric

- 1/4 tsp smoked paprika

- Salt and black pepper, to taste

- 2 large eggs (optional, for added protein)

- Optional toppings: Sliced avocado, hot sauce, or fresh parsley

Instructions

1. Cook the Sweet Potato:

- Heat 1 tablespoon of olive oil in a large skillet over medium heat.

- Add the sweet potato cubes and a pinch of salt. Sauté for 10-12 minutes, stirring occasionally, until the sweet potato starts to soften and develop a golden color.

2. Add Onion and Bell Pepper:

- Push the sweet potatoes to one side of the skillet and add the remaining tablespoon of oil.

- Add the diced onion and red bell pepper. Cook for 5-7 minutes, stirring occasionally, until the vegetables are tender.

3.   Add Kale and Spices:

•   Stir in the chopped kale, minced garlic, turmeric, smoked paprika, salt, and black pepper. Cook for 2-3 minutes, just until the kale wilts.

4.   Optional: Cook Eggs:

•   If adding eggs, create small wells in the hash and crack the eggs into them. Cover the skillet and cook for 3-4 minutes, or until the eggs are cooked to your desired doneness.

5.   Serve and Garnish:

•   Remove from heat and divide the hash onto plates. Add optional toppings like sliced avocado, hot sauce, or fresh parsley for extra flavor.

3. Blueberry Chia Pudding with Almond Milk

This simple and nutritious chia pudding is a fantastic anti-inflammatory breakfast or snack. Packed with antioxidants from blueberries and omega-3 fatty acids from chia seeds, it's a delicious way to support your body's fight against inflammation.

Ingredients (Serves 2)

•   1/2 cup chia seeds

•   1 cup unsweetened almond milk (or any milk of choice)

•   1/2 cup fresh or frozen blueberries

•   1 tsp maple syrup or honey (optional, for sweetness)

• 1/2 tsp vanilla extract

• 1/4 tsp ground cinnamon

• 1 tbsp almond butter (optional, for added creaminess)

• Optional toppings: Additional blueberries, shredded coconut, or sliced almonds

Instructions

1. Prepare the Chia Pudding:

• In a medium-sized bowl, combine the chia seeds, almond milk, maple syrup (if using), vanilla extract, and ground cinnamon. Stir well to ensure the chia seeds are evenly distributed.

2. Let It Set:

• Cover the bowl and refrigerate for at least 4 hours, or overnight, to allow the chia seeds to absorb the liquid and form a thick, pudding-like consistency. Stir once or twice during the first hour to prevent clumping.

3. Add Blueberries:

• Once the pudding has set, stir in the fresh or thawed frozen blueberries. If desired, mix in almond butter for added richness and creaminess.

4. Serve:

• Spoon the chia pudding into serving bowls or jars. Top with additional blueberries, sliced almonds, or shredded coconut for a finishing touch.

Why It's Anti-Inflammatory

• Chia Seeds: High in omega-3 fatty acids, which are known to reduce inflammation and support brain health.

• Blueberries: Packed with anthocyanins, antioxidants that combat oxidative stress and inflammation.

• Almond Milk: A dairy-free option that's low in saturated fat and supports heart health.

• Cinnamon: A spice that helps regulate blood sugar and reduces inflammation.

4. Spinach and Mushroom Omelette with Avocado

This nutrient-packed omelette is an excellent anti-inflammatory meal, combining the goodness of spinach, mushrooms, and avocado, all of which are known for their anti-inflammatory properties. It's a simple and satisfying breakfast or light lunch option.

Ingredients (Serves 1)

• 2 large eggs (or 3 egg whites + 1 whole egg for lower cholesterol)

• 1/2 cup fresh spinach, chopped

• 1/4 cup mushrooms, sliced

• 1/4 small onion, finely chopped

• 1/2 tbsp olive oil (or avocado oil)

• 1/2 ripe avocado, sliced

• Salt and black pepper, to taste

• 1/4 tsp turmeric (optional, for extra anti-inflammatory benefits)

• 1/4 tsp garlic powder (optional)

• Fresh parsley or chives, for garnish (optional)

Instructions

1. Sauté Vegetables:

• Heat the olive oil in a medium skillet over medium heat.

• Add the chopped onion and sliced mushrooms, and sauté for 3-4 minutes until softened.

• Add the spinach and cook for an additional 1-2 minutes until wilted. Optionally, sprinkle in turmeric and garlic powder for extra flavor and anti-inflammatory benefits. Remove the vegetables from the skillet and set them aside.

2. Prepare the Omelette:

• In a small bowl, whisk the eggs and season with salt and pepper.

• Pour the eggs into the same skillet and cook over low heat for about 1-2 minutes until the edges begin to set.

3. Fill the Omelette:

• Add the sautéed spinach and mushroom mixture to one half of the omelette. Let it cook for another 1-2 minutes, then fold the other side of the omelette over the filling.

4. Serve:

• Slide the omelette onto a plate and top with sliced avocado. Garnish with fresh parsley or chives if desired.

Why It's Anti-Inflammatory

• Spinach: Packed with anti-inflammatory compounds like flavonoids and antioxidants.

• Mushrooms: Rich in compounds like beta-glucans that boost immune function and fight inflammation.

• Avocado: Contains healthy fats (monounsaturated) and antioxidants that help reduce inflammation.

• Turmeric: Contains curcumin, a powerful anti-inflammatory agent.

• Olive Oil: Rich in oleocanthal, which works similarly to anti-inflammatory drugs.

5. Anti-Inflammatory Smoothie (Spinach, Pineapple, Ginger, Coconut Water)

This vibrant, nutrient-rich smoothie is designed to help fight inflammation while providing a refreshing and energizing boost. With the anti-inflammatory properties of spinach, pineapple, and ginger, combined with the hydrating benefits of coconut water, this smoothie is perfect for a post-workout recovery or a healthy snack.

Ingredients (Serves 2)

• 1 cup fresh spinach

• 1/2 cup frozen pineapple chunks

• 1/2 inch piece of fresh ginger, peeled and grated (or 1 tsp ground ginger)

• 1 cup coconut water

• 1/2 banana (for natural sweetness and creaminess)

• 1/2 tsp turmeric (optional, for an extra anti-inflammatory boost)

• Ice cubes (optional, for a colder texture)

• Optional add-ins: 1 tbsp chia seeds or flaxseeds, 1 tbsp coconut oil for added healthy fats

Instructions

1. Combine Ingredients:

• In a blender, add the spinach, pineapple, ginger, banana, and coconut water. If you're using turmeric or other add-ins, include them as well.

2. Blend:

• Blend on high until smooth, adding ice cubes if desired for a colder, thicker texture.

3. Taste and Adjust:

• Taste the smoothie and adjust sweetness if needed by adding a small amount of honey or maple syrup (optional). Blend again if needed.

4. Serve:

• Pour into glasses and serve immediately, garnished with a sprinkle of turmeric or a few pineapple chunks if desired.

Why It's Anti-Inflammatory

• Spinach: A rich source of antioxidants like flavonoids, which help reduce inflammation in the body.

• Pineapple: Contains bromelain, an enzyme with anti-inflammatory and digestive benefits.

• Ginger: Known for its powerful anti-inflammatory effects, ginger can help reduce swelling and promote overall health.

• Coconut Water: Hydrates the body and supports electrolyte balance, which is important for reducing inflammation.

• Turmeric: Contains curcumin, which is highly effective at combating inflammation.

6. Matcha Coconut Pancakes with Berries

These light and fluffy pancakes are packed with anti-inflammatory ingredients, including matcha, coconut, and antioxidant-rich berries. They make for a delightful breakfast or brunch option that's not only delicious but also supportive of your health.

Ingredients (Serves 2-3)

• 1/2 cup coconut flour

• 1/4 cup almond flour

• 1 tsp matcha powder (make sure it's high quality for maximum benefits)

• 1/2 tsp baking powder

• 1/4 tsp sea salt

• 3 large eggs

• 1/4 cup unsweetened coconut milk (or any milk of choice)

• 1 tbsp coconut oil, melted (plus extra for cooking)

• 1 tbsp honey (optional, for sweetness)

• 1/2 tsp vanilla extract

• Fresh mixed berries (e.g., blueberries, raspberries, strawberries) for topping

• Shredded coconut (optional, for garnish)

Instructions

1. Mix Dry Ingredients:

• In a large bowl, whisk together the coconut flour, almond flour, matcha powder, baking powder, and salt.

2. Prepare Wet Ingredients:

• In a separate bowl, whisk the eggs, coconut milk, melted coconut oil, honey, and vanilla extract until smooth.

3. Combine:

• Slowly pour the wet ingredients into the dry ingredients and stir until fully combined. The batter will be thick, but if it's too thick, add a little more coconut milk until you reach the desired consistency.

4. Cook the Pancakes:

• Heat a non-stick skillet or griddle over medium heat and lightly grease with coconut oil.

• Pour about 2-3 tbsp of batter per pancake onto the skillet, forming small rounds.

• Cook for 2-3 minutes on one side, or until bubbles start to form on the surface, then flip and cook for an additional 2-3 minutes until golden brown.

5. Serve:

• Stack the pancakes on a plate and top with fresh berries and a sprinkle of shredded coconut (if desired).

7. Quinoa Breakfast Bowl with Walnuts and Cinnamon

This warm and hearty breakfast bowl combines the protein-packed goodness of quinoa with the anti-inflammatory benefits of walnuts and cinnamon. It's a filling and satisfying meal that can be enjoyed any time of the day, while supporting your body with wholesome nutrients.

Ingredients (Serves 2)

- 1/2 cup quinoa (rinsed)

- 1 cup almond milk (or any milk of choice)

- 1/2 tsp ground cinnamon

- 1/4 tsp ground turmeric (optional, for added anti-inflammatory benefits)

- 1/2 tbsp honey (optional, for sweetness)

- 1/4 cup walnuts, chopped

- 1/4 cup dried cranberries or raisins (optional)

- Fresh fruit (e.g., berries, banana slices, or apple chunks)

- 1 tbsp chia seeds (optional, for added fiber and omega-3s)

Instructions

1. Cook Quinoa:

- In a medium saucepan, combine the rinsed quinoa and almond milk. Bring to a boil, then reduce the heat to low and cover.

- Let it simmer for 12-15 minutes until the quinoa is cooked and the liquid is absorbed. Fluff the quinoa with a fork.

2. Add Flavor:

• Stir in the ground cinnamon and turmeric (if using), and add honey for sweetness. Mix well.

3. Toast Walnuts:

• While the quinoa is cooking, toast the walnuts in a dry skillet over medium heat for 2-3 minutes until they are fragrant and lightly browned. Keep an eye on them to prevent burning.

4. Assemble the Bowl:

• Divide the cooked quinoa between two bowls. Top each bowl with toasted walnuts, dried cranberries (if using), chia seeds, and fresh fruit.

5. Serve:

• Enjoy warm for a comforting and anti-inflammatory breakfast!

Why It's Anti-Inflammatory

• Quinoa: A complete protein, quinoa is rich in fiber, magnesium, and antioxidants, which help reduce inflammation and support overall health.

• Walnuts: High in omega-3 fatty acids, walnuts have potent anti-inflammatory properties and promote heart health.

• Cinnamon: Contains cinnamaldehyde, a compound that has been shown to reduce inflammation and improve insulin sensitivity.

• Turmeric: Curcumin, the active compound in turmeric, is well-known for its powerful anti-inflammatory and antioxidant effects.

• Chia Seeds: Packed with fiber and omega-3 fatty acids, chia seeds help regulate inflammation and improve digestive health.

This Quinoa Breakfast Bowl with Walnuts and Cinnamon is a wholesome, delicious, and anti-inflammatory way to start your day. It's easily customizable with your favorite fruits, nuts, or seeds. Would you like more hearty breakfast options, or perhaps a savory bowl idea?

8. Baked Avocado Egg Cups

These Baked Avocado Egg Cups are a simple and nutritious breakfast or snack option, loaded with healthy fats and protein. The creamy avocado pairs perfectly with the baked egg, and it's naturally gluten-free, making it a great option for anyone following an anti-inflammatory diet.

Ingredients (Serves 2)

- 2 ripe avocados

- 4 large eggs

- Salt and pepper, to taste

- 1/4 tsp paprika (optional, for flavor)

- Fresh herbs (e.g., chives, parsley, or cilantro) for garnish

- Red pepper flakes (optional, for a bit of heat)

Instructions

1. Prepare the Avocados:

- Preheat your oven to 375°F (190°C).

- Cut the avocados in half and remove the pits. If the hole is too small to fit the egg, gently scoop out a bit of the flesh with a spoon to create a bigger space.

2. Bake the Avocados:

•   Place the avocado halves in a small baking dish or on a lined baking sheet.

•   Crack one egg into each avocado half. Be careful not to break the yolk. If needed, you can slightly adjust the avocado to level it so the egg stays in place.

3.   Season:

•   Sprinkle the eggs with salt, pepper, and paprika (if using).

4.   Bake:

•   Place the baking dish or sheet in the oven and bake for 12-15 minutes, or until the egg whites are set and the yolks are cooked to your desired consistency. For a runnier yolk, bake for less time.

5.   Serve:

•   Garnish with fresh herbs and a sprinkle of red pepper flakes, if desired. Serve immediately.

Why It's Anti-Inflammatory

•   Avocados: Rich in heart-healthy monounsaturated fats and antioxidants like vitamin E, avocados help reduce inflammation and promote overall health.

•   Eggs: A great source of high-quality protein and healthy fats, eggs contain essential nutrients like omega-3s (if using pasture-raised eggs), which have anti-inflammatory benefits.

•   Paprika: Contains capsaicin, which can help reduce inflammation and improve circulation.

•   Red Pepper Flakes: If included, the capsaicin in red pepper flakes has shown potential in reducing inflammatory markers in the body.

9. Banana Almond Butter Smoothie with Flaxseed

This creamy and satisfying smoothie combines the natural sweetness of bananas with the richness of almond butter and the fiber-packed goodness of flaxseed. It's a perfect breakfast or snack that supports inflammation reduction while providing a good balance of healthy fats, fiber, and antioxidants.

Ingredients (Serves 1)

- 1 ripe banana

- 1 tbsp almond butter (unsweetened)

- 1 tbsp flaxseed meal (ground)

- 1/2 cup unsweetened almond milk (or any milk of choice)

- 1/4 tsp cinnamon (optional, for extra flavor)

- 1-2 ice cubes (optional, for a colder, thicker texture)

- 1 tsp honey (optional, for added sweetness)

- 1/2 tsp vanilla extract (optional)

Instructions

1. Blend Ingredients:

- In a blender, combine the banana, almond butter, flaxseed meal, almond milk, cinnamon, and ice cubes (if using).

- Blend on high until smooth and creamy.

2. Adjust Consistency:

•   If the smoothie is too thick, add a bit more almond milk until it reaches your desired consistency.

3.   Sweeten:

•   If you prefer a sweeter smoothie, add the honey and vanilla extract, then blend again until fully combined.

4.   Serve:

•   Pour the smoothie into a glass and enjoy immediately.

Why It's Anti-Inflammatory

•   Bananas: Rich in potassium, fiber, and antioxidants, bananas help reduce inflammation and promote digestive health.

•   Almond Butter: A great source of healthy fats, particularly monounsaturated fats, almond butter helps support heart health and can reduce inflammation.

•   Flaxseed: Packed with omega-3 fatty acids, flaxseeds have potent anti-inflammatory properties and are also rich in fiber, supporting digestive health and helping regulate blood sugar.

•   Cinnamon: Known for its anti-inflammatory effects, cinnamon can help lower blood sugar and reduce oxidative stress.

•   Honey: A natural sweetener with antioxidant properties that may help reduce inflammation.

10. Ginger-Infused Oatmeal with Fresh Pears and Walnuts

This warm, comforting bowl of oatmeal is not only soothing but also packed with anti-inflammatory ingredients. The fresh pears add natural sweetness, while the walnuts provide healthy fats, and the ginger adds a spicy kick with inflammation-reducing benefits. Perfect for breakfast or a light, nourishing meal.

Ingredients (Serves 2)

- 1 cup rolled oats

- 2 cups water (or unsweetened almond milk for extra creaminess)

- 1 tsp fresh ginger, grated (or 1/2 tsp ground ginger)

- 1/2 tsp ground cinnamon

- 1/2 tsp turmeric (optional, for additional anti-inflammatory support)

- 1 medium pear, sliced

- 1/4 cup walnuts, chopped

- 1 tbsp chia seeds (optional, for added fiber and omega-3s)

- 1 tbsp honey or maple syrup (optional, for sweetness)

- Pinch of sea salt

- Fresh mint leaves (optional, for garnish)

Instructions

1. Prepare the Oats:

- In a medium saucepan, combine the rolled oats and water (or almond milk). Bring to a boil, then reduce the heat to low and simmer, stirring occasionally for about 5-7 minutes, or until the oats are soft and have absorbed most of the liquid.

2. Add Spices and Ginger:

• While the oats are cooking, stir in the grated ginger, cinnamon, turmeric (if using), and a pinch of sea salt. Stir well to incorporate the flavors.

3.   Assemble the Bowl:

• Once the oatmeal is cooked, divide it into two bowls. Top with sliced pears, chopped walnuts, chia seeds, and a drizzle of honey or maple syrup for sweetness.

4.   Garnish and Serve:

• Garnish with fresh mint leaves for an extra burst of flavor and color (optional). Serve immediately and enjoy!

Why It's Anti-Inflammatory

• Oats: Oats are rich in soluble fiber, particularly beta-glucan, which has been shown to help reduce cholesterol and inflammation in the body.

• Ginger: Ginger contains bioactive compounds like gingerol, which have potent anti-inflammatory and antioxidant properties. Ginger helps reduce muscle soreness, joint pain, and digestive discomfort.

• Pears: High in fiber and antioxidants, pears support gut health and help reduce oxidative stress, which is linked to chronic inflammation.

• Walnuts: Packed with omega-3 fatty acids, walnuts help fight inflammation and support heart health.

• Cinnamon: A powerful anti-inflammatory spice that can help reduce blood sugar levels and protect against oxidative stress.

• Turmeric: Contains curcumin, a compound known for its strong anti-inflammatory and antioxidant properties.

- Chia Seeds: Rich in omega-3 fatty acids, fiber, and antioxidants, chia seeds help reduce inflammation and support digestive and heart health.

Chapter 3
Wholesome Lunches (10 Recipes)

1. Quinoa Buddha Bowl with Roasted Veggies and Tahini Dressing

This vibrant, nutrient-packed Buddha bowl is a perfect example of an anti-inflammatory meal. The quinoa serves as a whole grain base, while the roasted vegetables add a rich array of antioxidants. Topped with a creamy, tangy tahini dressing, this dish is filling, balanced, and great for reducing inflammation.

Ingredients (Serves 2)

- 1 cup quinoa
- 2 cups water or vegetable broth
- 1 cup sweet potatoes, peeled and diced
- 1 cup Brussels sprouts, halved
- 1/2 cup red bell pepper, sliced
- 1/2 cup carrots, thinly sliced
- 1 tbsp olive oil
- Salt and pepper, to taste
- 1 tbsp sesame seeds (optional, for garnish)

- Fresh parsley or cilantro, chopped (for garnish)

For the Tahini Dressing

- 3 tbsp tahini

- 2 tbsp lemon juice

- 1 tbsp olive oil

- 1 tbsp water (or more for desired consistency)

- 1 garlic clove, minced

- 1 tsp maple syrup (optional, for sweetness)

- Salt and pepper, to taste

Instructions

1. Cook the Quinoa:

- Rinse the quinoa thoroughly under cold water. In a medium saucepan, bring the water or vegetable broth to a boil. Add the quinoa, reduce the heat to low, cover, and simmer for about 15 minutes, or until the quinoa is cooked and all the liquid is absorbed. Fluff with a fork and set aside.

2. Roast the Vegetables:

- Preheat your oven to 400°F (200°C).

- On a baking sheet, toss the diced sweet potatoes, Brussels sprouts, red bell pepper, and carrots with olive oil, salt, and pepper. Spread them out evenly and roast for about 20-25 minutes, or until the vegetables are tender and slightly caramelized, flipping halfway through.

3. Make the Tahini Dressing:

• In a small bowl, whisk together the tahini, lemon juice, olive oil, water, garlic, maple syrup (if using), and salt and pepper. Adjust the consistency by adding more water if needed. The dressing should be creamy and pourable.

4. Assemble the Buddha Bowl:

• Divide the cooked quinoa between two bowls. Top with the roasted vegetables, drizzle with the tahini dressing, and garnish with sesame seeds and fresh herbs.

5. Serve:

• Serve immediately as a wholesome, nourishing meal. Enjoy!

2. Wild-Caught Salmon Salad with Arugula and Pomegranate

This fresh and vibrant salad is packed with omega-3 fatty acids from wild-caught salmon, which are known for their powerful anti-inflammatory properties. The peppery arugula and sweet pomegranate seeds create a delicious balance of flavors, while the citrusy dressing adds a zesty kick. Perfect for lunch or a light dinner, this salad is as nourishing as it is flavorful.

Ingredients (Serves 2)

• 2 wild-caught salmon fillets (about 4-6 oz each)

• 4 cups arugula (fresh)

• 1/2 cup pomegranate seeds

- 1/4 cup walnuts, chopped

- 1/4 cup red onion, thinly sliced

- 1/2 avocado, sliced

- Olive oil, for cooking

- Salt and pepper, to taste

For the Dressing

- 2 tbsp olive oil

- 1 tbsp balsamic vinegar

- 1 tbsp fresh lemon juice

- 1 tsp Dijon mustard

- 1 tsp honey (optional, for sweetness)

- Salt and pepper, to taste

Instructions

1. Cook the Salmon:

- Heat a small amount of olive oil in a pan over medium heat.

- Season the salmon fillets with salt and pepper.

- Place the salmon in the pan, skin side down if it has skin, and cook for about 4-5 minutes on each side, or until it is cooked through and easily flakes with a fork. Remove from the heat and set aside to cool slightly.

2. Prepare the Salad:

- While the salmon is cooking, arrange the arugula, pomegranate seeds, walnuts, red onion, and avocado slices in a large salad bowl.

3. Make the Dressing:

• In a small bowl, whisk together the olive oil, balsamic vinegar, lemon juice, Dijon mustard, honey (if using), salt, and pepper until well combined.

4. Assemble the Salad:

• Flake the salmon into large chunks and add it to the salad bowl.

• Drizzle the dressing over the salad and toss gently to combine.

5. Serve:

• Serve immediately as a light yet satisfying meal.

3. Lentil and Sweet Potato Stew

This hearty and comforting stew is packed with plant-based protein from lentils, anti-inflammatory compounds from sweet potatoes, and a rich variety of spices. The combination of fiber, antioxidants, and healthy carbohydrates makes this a perfect meal to promote gut health and reduce inflammation. This stew is also great for meal prep as it stores well and tastes even better the next day.

Ingredients (Serves 4-6)

• 1 cup dried green or brown lentils, rinsed

• 2 medium sweet potatoes, peeled and diced

• 1 onion, chopped

• 2 garlic cloves, minced

- 2 carrots, diced

- 2 celery stalks, chopped

- 1 can (14.5 oz) diced tomatoes (with juices)

- 4 cups vegetable broth (or water)

- 1 tsp turmeric

- 1 tsp cumin

- 1/2 tsp ground coriander

- 1/2 tsp smoked paprika

- 1/4 tsp cayenne pepper (optional, for heat)

- 1 tbsp olive oil

- Salt and pepper, to taste

- 2 cups spinach (fresh or frozen)

- Juice of 1 lemon

- Fresh parsley, chopped (for garnish)

Instructions

1. Prepare the Base:

- In a large pot, heat the olive oil over medium heat. Add the chopped onion, garlic, carrots, and celery. Sauté for about 5-7 minutes, or until the vegetables start to soften and the onion is translucent.

2. Add the Spices:

- Add the turmeric, cumin, coriander, smoked paprika, and cayenne pepper (if using). Stir the mixture for about 1-2 minutes, allowing the spices to become fragrant.

3.   Add the Lentils and Sweet Potatoes:

•   Add the rinsed lentils, diced sweet potatoes, and diced tomatoes to the pot. Stir to combine with the aromatic vegetables and spices.

4.   Simmer the Stew:

•   Pour in the vegetable broth (or water) and bring to a boil. Reduce the heat to low, cover, and simmer for about 30-40 minutes, or until the lentils are tender and the sweet potatoes are cooked through. Stir occasionally and add more water if needed to reach your desired consistency.

5.   Finish the Stew:

•   Once the lentils and sweet potatoes are cooked, stir in the spinach and cook for an additional 3-5 minutes, until wilted (if using fresh spinach). Season with salt and pepper to taste.

6.   Serve:

•   Squeeze fresh lemon juice over the stew for added brightness and garnish with fresh parsley. Serve hot with a side of whole grain bread or over brown rice, if desired.

4.   Mediterranean Chickpea Salad with Lemon and Olive Oil

This vibrant and refreshing salad is packed with anti-inflammatory ingredients like chickpeas, olive oil, and fresh vegetables. The Mediterranean diet is known for its focus on healthy fats, fiber, and antioxidants, which help combat inflammation and support overall health. This salad is perfect for a light lunch, side dish, or as a meal prep option.

Ingredients (Serves 4)

- 2 cans (15 oz each) chickpeas, drained and rinsed

- 1 cucumber, diced

- 1 pint cherry tomatoes, halved

- 1/4 red onion, thinly sliced

- 1/4 cup Kalamata olives, pitted and sliced

- 1/4 cup fresh parsley, chopped

- 1/4 cup feta cheese, crumbled (optional)

- 2 tbsp extra virgin olive oil

- 1 tbsp lemon juice (freshly squeezed)

- 1 tsp dried oregano

- 1/2 tsp garlic powder

- Salt and pepper, to taste

Instructions

1. Prepare the Ingredients:

- In a large bowl, combine the chickpeas, diced cucumber, halved cherry tomatoes, sliced red onion, Kalamata olives, and chopped parsley.

2. Make the Dressing:

- In a small bowl, whisk together the olive oil, lemon juice, dried oregano, garlic powder, salt, and pepper until well combined.

3.   Toss the Salad:

•   Pour the dressing over the salad and toss everything together gently until the ingredients are evenly coated.

4.   Add Feta (Optional):

•   If using feta cheese, sprinkle it over the top of the salad for added flavor and texture.

5.   Serve:

•   Serve immediately as a refreshing side dish or main meal. This salad also keeps well in the refrigerator for up to 2-3 days, making it perfect for meal prep.

5.   Zucchini Noodles with Pesto and Grilled Chicken

This healthy, low-carb, anti-inflammatory meal is packed with fresh zucchini, flavorful pesto, and lean grilled chicken. Zucchini noodles are a great alternative to pasta, offering more nutrients and fiber while being gentle on the digestive system. The addition of pesto provides a rich source of healthy fats from olive oil, and the grilled chicken gives a boost of lean protein. This meal is perfect for lunch or dinner and helps support inflammation reduction and overall wellness.

Ingredients (Serves 4)

•   4 medium zucchinis, spiralized into noodles (or use a vegetable peeler to create ribbons)

•   2 chicken breasts, boneless and skinless

- 2 tbsp olive oil

- 1 tsp garlic powder

- Salt and pepper, to taste

For the Pesto:

- 1 cup fresh basil leaves

- 1/4 cup pine nuts (or walnuts for a different flavor)

- 1/4 cup Parmesan cheese, grated (optional for dairy-free version)

- 2 cloves garlic, minced

- 1/4 cup extra virgin olive oil

- 1 tbsp lemon juice

- 1/2 tsp salt

- 1/4 tsp black pepper

Instructions

1. Prepare the Chicken:

- Preheat a grill or grill pan over medium heat.

- Rub the chicken breasts with 1 tablespoon of olive oil, garlic powder, salt, and pepper.

- Grill the chicken for 6-7 minutes per side, or until the internal temperature reaches 165°F (74°C). Once cooked, remove from the grill and let rest before slicing into strips.

2. Make the Pesto:

• In a food processor, combine the basil, pine nuts, Parmesan cheese (if using), garlic, olive oil, lemon juice, salt, and pepper. Pulse until smooth, scraping down the sides as needed. Adjust seasoning to taste, adding more lemon juice or salt if necessary.

3. Prepare the Zucchini Noodles:

• Using a spiralizer, vegetable peeler, or mandoline, create zucchini noodles. If you don't have a spiralizer, you can also use a regular vegetable peeler to create zucchini ribbons.

4. Sauté the Zucchini Noodles:

• In a large skillet, heat the remaining 1 tablespoon of olive oil over medium heat. Add the zucchini noodles and sauté for 2-3 minutes, or until just tender. Be careful not to overcook them, as zucchini can release excess water and become mushy.

5. Assemble the Dish:

• Toss the zucchini noodles with the pesto, ensuring the noodles are well-coated.

• Serve the pesto zucchini noodles topped with sliced grilled chicken.

6. Serve:

• Garnish with extra basil, pine nuts, or grated Parmesan if desired. Serve immediately and enjoy!

6.   Turmeric-Spiced Cauliflower Soup

This warm, comforting soup is packed with anti-inflammatory goodness from cauliflower, turmeric, and other spices. Cauliflower is a versatile vegetable that is rich in fiber, antioxidants, and vitamins. When paired with turmeric, known for its potent anti-inflammatory compound curcumin, this soup becomes a powerful meal for reducing inflammation and supporting overall health. This easy-to-make, vegan-friendly soup is perfect for lunch or dinner, especially on colder days.

Ingredients (Serves 4-6)

- 1 large head of cauliflower, cut into florets

- 1 medium onion, chopped

- 2 cloves garlic, minced

- 1 tsp ground turmeric

- 1 tsp ground cumin

- 1/2 tsp ground coriander

- 1/4 tsp ground black pepper (to enhance turmeric absorption)

- 4 cups vegetable broth (low-sodium)

- 1 cup coconut milk (or almond milk for a lighter version)

- 2 tbsp olive oil

- 1 tbsp fresh ginger, grated

- 1 tbsp lemon juice

- Salt, to taste

- Fresh cilantro, for garnish (optional)

- Crumbled roasted almonds or cashews, for garnish (optional)

Instructions

1. Sauté the Aromatics:

• In a large pot, heat the olive oil over medium heat.

• Add the chopped onion and sauté for 5-7 minutes, or until the onion becomes soft and translucent.

• Add the minced garlic, grated ginger, turmeric, cumin, coriander, and black pepper. Stir well to coat the onions and garlic in the spices, cooking for 1-2 minutes to release the aromas.

2. Cook the Cauliflower:

• Add the cauliflower florets to the pot, stirring to combine with the aromatics and spices.

• Pour in the vegetable broth, ensuring the cauliflower is covered by the liquid. Bring to a boil, then reduce the heat to a simmer.

• Let the soup simmer for 15-20 minutes, or until the cauliflower is tender and can be easily pierced with a fork.

3. Blend the Soup:

• Once the cauliflower is tender, remove the pot from the heat.

• Use an immersion blender to blend the soup until smooth and creamy. If you don't have an immersion blender, carefully transfer the soup in batches to a regular blender and blend until smooth.

• For a thicker soup, leave some chunks of cauliflower, or for a smoother texture, blend until completely creamy.

4. Add Coconut Milk and Lemon:

• Stir in the coconut milk and lemon juice. Taste and adjust seasoning, adding salt as needed.

5. Serve:

• Ladle the soup into bowls and garnish with fresh cilantro and crumbled roasted almonds or cashews for added texture and flavor.

6.   Enjoy:

•   Serve this warm and nourishing soup with a side of whole-grain bread or a light salad for a complete meal.

7.   Avocado and Hummus Wrap with Spinach and Cucumber

This refreshing and easy-to-make wrap is packed with healthy fats from avocado, fiber and protein from hummus, and a boost of vitamins and minerals from fresh spinach and cucumber. The combination of these anti-inflammatory ingredients creates a balanced meal that's both satisfying and nutritious. It's perfect for a light lunch or a quick snack and can be made in just a few minutes.

Ingredients (Serves 2)

•   2 whole wheat or gluten-free wraps (or any preferred wrap)

•   1 ripe avocado, sliced

•   1/2 cup hummus (store-bought or homemade)

•   1 cup fresh spinach leaves

•   1/2 cucumber, thinly sliced

•   1 tbsp olive oil (optional, for drizzling)

•   Juice of 1/2 lemon

•   Salt and pepper, to taste

•   1/4 tsp ground paprika (optional, for extra flavor)

Instructions

1. Prepare the Ingredients:

•   Slice the avocado into thin wedges.

•   Thinly slice the cucumber and set aside.

•   Wash and dry the spinach leaves.

2. Assemble the Wrap:

•   Lay the whole wheat or gluten-free wraps flat on a clean surface.

•   Spread 1/4 cup of hummus evenly on each wrap, leaving about an inch from the edges.

•   Place a handful of fresh spinach leaves in the center of each wrap.

•   Arrange the avocado slices and cucumber slices on top of the spinach.

3. Season and Drizzle:

•   Drizzle the wraps with a little olive oil, if desired.

•   Squeeze lemon juice over the veggies and avocado, and season with salt, pepper, and a sprinkle of paprika for extra flavor.

4. Roll the Wrap:

•   Carefully fold the sides of the wrap inwards, then roll it tightly from the bottom up to secure the ingredients.

5. Serve:

•   Slice the wrap in half at a diagonal and serve immediately.

6. Enjoy:

• Enjoy this fresh and anti-inflammatory wrap as a quick lunch or snack on the go!

8. Miso Soup with Tofu, Wakame, and Green Onions

This soothing, savory miso soup is not only comforting but also packed with anti-inflammatory ingredients that promote gut health and overall well-being. Miso, a fermented food, contains probiotics that support gut health, while tofu provides plant-based protein. Wakame (seaweed) is rich in minerals and antioxidants, and green onions add a fresh, mild flavor. This soup is perfect as a light meal or as an appetizer to complement a larger anti-inflammatory meal.

Ingredients (Serves 4)

• 4 cups water

• 2 tbsp miso paste (preferably organic, and choose either white or red miso based on your preference)

• 200g firm tofu, cut into cubes

• 1/4 cup dried wakame seaweed

• 2 green onions, chopped

• 1-2 tsp tamari or soy sauce (optional, for added umami flavor)

• 1 tbsp rice vinegar (optional, for extra tanginess)

• 1 tsp sesame oil (optional, for extra flavor)

- 1 tsp grated fresh ginger (optional, for an added anti-inflammatory boost)

- 1/2 tsp garlic powder (optional)

Instructions

1. Rehydrate the Wakame:

- In a small bowl, place the dried wakame and cover it with warm water. Let it soak for about 5-10 minutes to rehydrate, then drain and set aside.

2. Prepare the Broth:

- In a medium-sized pot, bring the 4 cups of water to a simmer over medium heat.

- Once the water is hot, add the miso paste and stir well to dissolve it completely into the water. Continue to heat the broth, but do not allow it to boil.

- Add the tamari or soy sauce (if using), rice vinegar (optional), and grated ginger for extra flavor.

3. Add Tofu and Wakame:

- Gently add the cubed tofu and rehydrated wakame to the pot. Let the mixture simmer for 2-3 minutes to warm the tofu and allow the flavors to meld together.

4. Garnish and Serve:

- Stir in the chopped green onions and drizzle the sesame oil over the soup (optional).

- Taste and adjust seasoning, adding garlic powder or additional soy sauce if desired.

5. Serve:

• Ladle the soup into bowls and enjoy immediately while hot.

9. Grilled Shrimp Tacos with Mango Salsa

These grilled shrimp tacos are light, flavorful, and packed with anti-inflammatory ingredients. The shrimp provides lean protein, while the mango salsa adds a sweet and tangy twist with anti-inflammatory benefits from ingredients like cilantro and lime. Served in corn tortillas, these tacos are perfect for a healthy, delicious meal that supports your body's inflammation response.

Ingredients (Serves 4)

For the Grilled Shrimp:

• 1 lb shrimp, peeled and deveined

• 1 tbsp olive oil

• 1 tsp chili powder

• 1/2 tsp cumin

• 1/4 tsp turmeric (anti-inflammatory)

• 1/2 tsp garlic powder

• 1/4 tsp smoked paprika

• Salt and pepper, to taste

• Juice of 1 lime

For the Mango Salsa:

- 1 ripe mango, diced

- 1/4 red onion, finely chopped

- 1/2 red bell pepper, diced

- 1/2 cucumber, diced

- 1/4 cup fresh cilantro, chopped

- 1 tbsp lime juice

- Salt and pepper, to taste

For Assembly:

- 8 small corn tortillas (or gluten-free tortillas)

- 1 avocado, sliced (optional, for added creaminess)

- Lime wedges, for serving

Instructions

1. Prepare the Shrimp Marinade:

- In a bowl, combine olive oil, chili powder, cumin, turmeric, garlic powder, smoked paprika, salt, pepper, and lime juice.

- Add the shrimp and toss until well coated. Let marinate for at least 15-20 minutes to allow the flavors to meld.

2. Make the Mango Salsa:

- In a separate bowl, combine diced mango, red onion, red bell pepper, cucumber, and fresh cilantro.

- Add lime juice, salt, and pepper to taste. Stir gently and set aside to allow the flavors to develop.

3. Grill the Shrimp:

- Preheat your grill or grill pan to medium-high heat.

- Thread the marinated shrimp onto skewers or place directly on the grill. Grill for 2-3 minutes per side until the shrimp are opaque and cooked through.

4. Warm the Tortillas:

- While the shrimp is grilling, heat the tortillas on the grill or in a dry skillet for 30 seconds per side until warm and slightly charred.

5. Assemble the Tacos:

- Place the grilled shrimp on the warm tortillas.

- Top with a generous spoonful of mango salsa and slices of avocado, if desired.

- Serve with lime wedges on the side for extra zest.

6. Serve and Enjoy:

- Serve the tacos immediately while warm, and enjoy the fresh, vibrant flavors!

10. Spaghetti Squash with Tomato Basil Sauce

This dish is a nutrient-packed, anti-inflammatory alternative to traditional pasta. Spaghetti squash, when roasted, naturally separates into tender strands resembling spaghetti, making it a great low-carb, gluten-free option. Paired with a simple, fresh tomato basil sauce, this meal is rich in antioxidants and anti-inflammatory compounds, perfect for anyone looking to reduce inflammation while enjoying a delicious meal.

Ingredients (Serves 4)

For the Spaghetti Squash:

- 1 medium spaghetti squash
- 1 tbsp olive oil
- Salt and pepper, to taste

For the Tomato Basil Sauce:

- 2 tbsp olive oil
- 1 small onion, finely chopped
- 4 garlic cloves, minced
- 1 can (14.5 oz) crushed tomatoes (preferably no added sugar)
- 1/4 cup fresh basil, chopped
- 1/2 tsp dried oregano
- 1/4 tsp red pepper flakes (optional for a little heat)
- Salt and pepper, to taste
- 1 tbsp balsamic vinegar (optional for extra depth of flavor)

For Garnish (optional):

- Fresh basil leaves, for garnish
- Grated Parmesan or dairy-free cheese, for serving (optional)

Instructions

1. Prepare the Spaghetti Squash:

- Preheat the oven to 400°F (200°C).

- Slice the spaghetti squash in half lengthwise and scoop out the seeds.

- Drizzle the cut sides with olive oil, then season with salt and pepper.

- Place the squash halves, cut-side down, on a baking sheet lined with parchment paper.

- Roast in the oven for 40-45 minutes, or until the squash is tender and easily pierced with a fork.

- Once cooked, use a fork to scrape the flesh, which will naturally separate into spaghetti-like strands.

2. Make the Tomato Basil Sauce:

- While the squash is roasting, heat 2 tbsp olive oil in a large skillet over medium heat.

- Add the chopped onion and sauté for about 5 minutes until softened.

- Add the minced garlic and cook for an additional 1-2 minutes until fragrant.

- Stir in the crushed tomatoes, basil, oregano, red pepper flakes (if using), and balsamic vinegar (if using).

- Simmer the sauce for 10-15 minutes, allowing the flavors to meld and the sauce to thicken.

- Season with salt and pepper to taste.

3. Combine and Serve:

- Once the spaghetti squash is ready, use a fork to scrape out the strands and place them in a large serving bowl.

- Pour the tomato basil sauce over the squash and toss to combine.

- Garnish with fresh basil and top with grated cheese (if desired).

4. Serve:

- Serve warm and enjoy this healthy, anti-inflammatory meal!

Chapter 4

Nourishing Dinners (10 Recipes)

1. Herb-Crusted Cod with Asparagus and Lemon

Ingredients:

- 4 cod fillets (about 6 ounces each)

- 1 pound asparagus, trimmed

- 2 tablespoons olive oil, divided

- 1 lemon, thinly sliced (plus extra for garnish)

- 1/2 cup breadcrumbs (panko works best)

- 1/4 cup Parmesan cheese, grated

- 2 tablespoons fresh parsley, finely chopped

- 1 teaspoon garlic powder

- 1 teaspoon dried thyme

- Salt and pepper, to taste

- Lemon wedges (for serving)

Instructions:

1. Preheat the oven:

Preheat your oven to 400°F (200°C). Line a baking sheet with parchment paper or foil for easy cleanup.

2. Prepare the asparagus:

Place the asparagus on one side of the baking sheet. Drizzle with 1 tablespoon of olive oil, sprinkle with salt and pepper, and toss to coat. Lay the lemon slices over the asparagus.

3. Make the herb crust:

In a small bowl, combine breadcrumbs, Parmesan cheese, parsley, garlic powder, thyme, a pinch of salt, and pepper. Add 1 tablespoon of olive oil and mix until the crumbs are evenly coated and slightly moist.

4. Season the cod:

Pat the cod fillets dry with paper towels and place them on the other side of the baking sheet. Lightly season with salt and pepper.

5. Add the crust:

Press the breadcrumb mixture onto the top of each cod fillet, ensuring an even layer.

6. Bake:

Place the baking sheet in the preheated oven and bake for 12-15 minutes, or until the cod is opaque and flakes easily with a fork, and the asparagus is tender-crisp.

7. Broil (optional):

For a golden crust, switch the oven to broil for the last 2-3 minutes of cooking. Watch closely to avoid burning.

8. Serve:

Remove from the oven and serve immediately, garnished with fresh parsley and lemon wedges for extra flavor.

2. Grass-Fed Beef Stir-Fry with Ginger and Broccoli

Ingredients:

*   1 pound grass-fed beef sirloin or flank steak, thinly sliced against the grain

*   2 tablespoons soy sauce (or tamari for gluten-free)

*   1 tablespoon cornstarch (or arrowroot powder)

*   1 tablespoon rice vinegar

*   1 tablespoon sesame oil, divided

*   1 tablespoon olive oil

*   1 tablespoon fresh ginger, minced

*   3 cloves garlic, minced

*   4 cups broccoli florets

*   1 red bell pepper, thinly sliced

*   1/4 cup water or beef broth

*   2 tablespoons oyster sauce (optional, for added depth)

*   1 teaspoon honey or maple syrup (optional, for a touch of sweetness)

*   Sesame seeds and green onions, for garnish

*   Steamed rice or noodles, for serving

Instructions:

1.   Marinate the beef:

In a medium bowl, combine soy sauce, cornstarch, and rice vinegar. Add the beef slices, toss to coat, and let marinate for 10-15 minutes.

2.   Prepare the sauce:

In a small bowl, mix oyster sauce (if using), honey, and 1/4 cup water or broth. Set aside.

3.   Cook the beef:

Heat a large skillet or wok over medium-high heat. Add 1/2 tablespoon sesame oil and the olive oil. Once hot, add the beef in a single layer. Sear for 1-2 minutes per side until browned. Remove the beef and set aside.

4.   Cook the vegetables:

In the same skillet, add the remaining sesame oil. Sauté ginger and garlic for 30 seconds until fragrant. Add broccoli and red bell pepper. Stir-fry for 2-3 minutes, then add the water or broth. Cover and steam for 2-3 minutes until the broccoli is tender-crisp.

5.   Combine everything:

Return the beef to the skillet. Pour in the prepared sauce and toss to combine. Cook for 1-2 minutes until the sauce thickens slightly and coats the beef and vegetables.

6.   Serve:

Transfer to a serving platter or bowl. Garnish with sesame seeds and sliced green onions. Serve hot over steamed rice or noodles.

This flavorful stir-fry is packed with protein and nutrients, perfect for a quick and healthy meal!

3. Baked Eggplant with Spiced Tomato Sauce and Fresh Basil

Ingredients:

For the Eggplant:

- 2 medium eggplants, sliced into 1/2-inch rounds
- 1 tablespoon salt (for draining)
- 2 tablespoons olive oil
- 1/2 teaspoon garlic powder
- 1/4 teaspoon black pepper

For the Spiced Tomato Sauce:

- 1 tablespoon olive oil
- 1 medium onion, finely chopped
- 3 garlic cloves, minced
- 1 teaspoon ground cumin
- 1 teaspoon smoked paprika
- 1/2 teaspoon red pepper flakes (optional, for heat)
- 1 (14-ounce) can diced tomatoes or crushed tomatoes
- 1/2 teaspoon sugar (to balance acidity)
- Salt and pepper, to taste

For Assembly:

- 1/2 cup mozzarella cheese, shredded (optional)

- 1/4 cup Parmesan cheese, grated

- Fresh basil leaves, for garnish

Instructions:

1. Prepare the Eggplant:

1.   Arrange the eggplant slices on a large baking sheet lined with paper towels. Sprinkle both sides generously with salt and let sit for 20-30 minutes to draw out excess moisture and bitterness.

2.   Rinse the eggplant slices under cold water and pat them dry with a clean kitchen towel.

3.   Preheat your oven to 400°F (200°C). Arrange the eggplant slices on a parchment-lined baking sheet. Brush both sides with olive oil and sprinkle with garlic powder and black pepper.

4.   Bake for 20-25 minutes, flipping halfway, until the eggplant is golden and tender.

2. Make the Spiced Tomato Sauce:

1.   Heat olive oil in a medium saucepan over medium heat. Add the chopped onion and sauté for 3-4 minutes until softened.

2.   Stir in the garlic, cumin, smoked paprika, and red pepper flakes (if using). Cook for 30 seconds until fragrant.

3.   Add the diced tomatoes and sugar. Simmer for 10-15 minutes, stirring occasionally, until the sauce thickens. Season with salt and pepper to taste.

3. Assemble and Bake:

1.   Reduce oven temperature to 375°F (190°C).

2.   Spread a thin layer of the tomato sauce in the bottom of a baking dish. Arrange a layer of baked eggplant slices on top. Repeat with remaining sauce and eggplant, finishing with a layer of sauce.

3.   If using cheese, sprinkle the mozzarella and Parmesan over the top.

4.   Bake uncovered for 15-20 minutes, until the cheese is melted and bubbling.

4. Serve:

1.   Remove from the oven and let cool slightly. Garnish with fresh basil leaves.

2.   Serve warm as a main dish or side, paired with crusty bread or a fresh salad.

This dish is rich in Mediterranean flavors and perfect for a hearty vegetarian meal!

4.   Coconut Curry with Chickpeas and Spinach

Ingredients:

- 1 tablespoon olive oil
- 1 medium onion, finely chopped
- 3 garlic cloves, minced
- 1 tablespoon fresh ginger, grated
- 2 tablespoons red curry paste (adjust for spice level)
- 1 teaspoon ground turmeric

- 1/2 teaspoon ground cumin

- 1 (14-ounce) can coconut milk (full-fat or light)

- 1 (14-ounce) can diced tomatoes

- 1 (14-ounce) can chickpeas, drained and rinsed

- 4 cups fresh spinach (or 1 bag baby spinach)

- 1 tablespoon soy sauce (or tamari for gluten-free)

- 1 teaspoon sugar (optional, to balance flavors)

- Salt and pepper, to taste

- Juice of 1/2 lime

- Fresh cilantro, for garnish

- Cooked rice or naan, for serving

Instructions:

1. Sauté the Aromatics:

    1. Heat olive oil in a large skillet or pot over medium heat.

    2. Add the onion and sauté for 3-4 minutes until softened.

    3. Stir in the garlic and ginger, cooking for 1 minute until fragrant.

2. Build the Curry Base:

    1. Add the red curry paste, turmeric, and cumin. Stir well to combine with the onion mixture and cook for 1 minute to enhance the flavors.

    2. Pour in the coconut milk and diced tomatoes. Stir to blend everything together.

3. Simmer:

    1.   Bring the mixture to a gentle simmer. Add the chickpeas and let it cook for 8-10 minutes, allowing the flavors to meld and the sauce to thicken slightly.

4. Add Spinach:

    1.   Stir in the spinach and cook for 2-3 minutes until it wilts.

    2.   Add the soy sauce, sugar (if using), and lime juice. Taste and adjust with salt and pepper as needed.

5. Serve:

    1.   Spoon the curry over cooked rice or serve with naan bread.

    2.   Garnish with fresh cilantro and a squeeze of lime for extra brightness.

This hearty, plant-based dish is quick to prepare and packed with creamy, spiced flavor!

5.   Grilled Chicken with Quinoa Pilaf and Steamed Green Beans

Ingredients:

For the Grilled Chicken:

- 4 boneless, skinless chicken breasts

- 2 tablespoons olive oil

- 1 teaspoon garlic powder

- 1 teaspoon smoked paprika

- 1/2 teaspoon dried oregano

- Salt and pepper, to taste

- Juice of 1/2 lemon

For the Quinoa Pilaf:

- 1 cup quinoa, rinsed

- 2 cups chicken or vegetable broth

- 1 tablespoon olive oil

- 1 small onion, finely chopped

- 1 garlic clove, minced

- 1/2 cup diced carrots

- 1/2 cup frozen peas

- 1/4 cup chopped fresh parsley

- Salt and pepper, to taste

For the Steamed Green Beans:

- 1 pound fresh green beans, trimmed

- 1 tablespoon butter or olive oil

- Salt and pepper, to taste

- Lemon wedges, for serving

Instructions:

1. Marinate the Chicken:

1. In a small bowl, mix olive oil, garlic powder, smoked paprika, oregano, salt, pepper, and lemon juice.

2. Rub the mixture over the chicken breasts. Cover and let marinate for 20-30 minutes.

2. Cook the Quinoa Pilaf:

1. Heat olive oil in a medium saucepan over medium heat. Add the onion and sauté for 3-4 minutes until softened.

2. Stir in garlic and cook for 30 seconds. Add carrots and cook for another 2 minutes.

3. Add the quinoa and broth. Bring to a boil, then reduce heat to low, cover, and simmer for 15 minutes or until the liquid is absorbed.

4. Stir in peas and parsley, then season with salt and pepper. Set aside, covered.

3. Grill the Chicken:

1. Preheat a grill or grill pan over medium-high heat. Lightly oil the grates to prevent sticking.

2. Grill the chicken for 5-7 minutes per side, or until the internal temperature reaches 165°F (75°C). Remove and let rest for 5 minutes.

4. Steam the Green Beans:

1. Bring a pot of water to a boil and place a steamer basket over it. Add green beans, cover, and steam for 5-7 minutes until tender-crisp.

2. Toss with butter or olive oil and season with salt and pepper.

5. Assemble and Serve:

1. Plate the grilled chicken alongside the quinoa pilaf and green beans.

2. Serve with lemon wedges for a fresh squeeze of flavor.

This balanced and nutritious meal is flavorful, satisfying, and perfect for any occasion!

6. Stuffed Bell Peppers with Turkey, Black Beans, and Brown Rice

Ingredients:

- 6 large bell peppers (any color, tops removed, seeds and membranes cleaned)

- 1 tablespoon olive oil

- 1 pound ground turkey

- 1 small onion, finely chopped

- 3 garlic cloves, minced

- 1 teaspoon ground cumin

- 1 teaspoon smoked paprika

- 1/2 teaspoon chili powder (optional, for heat)

- 1 (14-ounce) can black beans, drained and rinsed

- 1 cup cooked brown rice

- 1 (14-ounce) can diced tomatoes, drained

- 1 cup shredded cheese (cheddar, Monterey Jack, or a blend)

- Salt and pepper, to taste

- Fresh cilantro, for garnish (optional)

Instructions:

1. Prepare the Bell Peppers:

    1.   Preheat your oven to 375°F (190°C).

    2.   Arrange the bell peppers upright in a baking dish. If necessary, trim the bottoms slightly to help them stand.

2. Cook the Filling:

    1.   Heat olive oil in a large skillet over medium heat. Add the onion and sauté for 3-4 minutes until softened.

    2.   Add the garlic and cook for 30 seconds until fragrant.

    3.   Stir in the ground turkey, breaking it into small pieces. Cook until browned and no longer pink, about 5-7 minutes.

    4.   Season with cumin, smoked paprika, chili powder (if using), salt, and pepper. Mix well.

    5.   Stir in the black beans, cooked brown rice, and diced tomatoes. Cook for 2-3 minutes until heated through.

3. Stuff the Peppers:

    1.   Spoon the turkey mixture into each bell pepper, packing it tightly.

    2.   Sprinkle shredded cheese on top of each pepper.

4. Bake:

    1.   Cover the baking dish with foil and bake for 25 minutes.

    2.   Remove the foil and bake for an additional 10-15 minutes, or until the peppers are tender and the cheese is melted and bubbly.

5. Serve:

    1.   Remove from the oven and let cool slightly.

    2.   Garnish with fresh cilantro, if desired, and serve warm.

These stuffed peppers are a hearty, protein-packed meal that's perfect for meal prep or a family dinner!

7.   Lemon-Dill Baked Salmon with Garlic Spinach

Ingredients:

For the Salmon:

- 4 salmon fillets (about 6 ounces each)

- 2 tablespoons olive oil

- 2 tablespoons fresh dill, chopped (or 1 teaspoon dried dill)

- 2 garlic cloves, minced

- 1 lemon, thinly sliced

- Salt and pepper, to taste

For the Garlic Spinach:

- 1 tablespoon olive oil

- 3 garlic cloves, minced

- 8 cups fresh spinach (about 2 large bunches)

- 1/2 teaspoon salt

- 1/4 teaspoon black pepper

- Juice of 1/2 lemon

Instructions:

1. Prepare the Salmon:

   1. Preheat your oven to 375°F (190°C). Line a baking sheet with parchment paper or lightly grease it.

   2. Place the salmon fillets on the baking sheet, skin side down if applicable.

   3. Drizzle the olive oil over the salmon, then sprinkle with dill, minced garlic, salt, and pepper.

   4. Arrange the lemon slices on top of the salmon fillets.

2. Bake the Salmon:

   1. Bake the salmon in the preheated oven for 12-15 minutes, or until the salmon flakes easily with a fork and reaches an internal temperature of 145°F (63°C).

3. Cook the Garlic Spinach:

   1. While the salmon is baking, heat olive oil in a large skillet over medium heat.

   2. Add the minced garlic and sauté for 1 minute until fragrant.

   3. Add the spinach in batches, stirring until wilted. This should take about 2-3 minutes.

   4. Season with salt, pepper, and a squeeze of lemon juice. Stir to combine, then remove from heat.

4. Serve:

1.   Plate the baked salmon alongside the garlic spinach.

2.   Optionally garnish with extra fresh dill and serve with lemon wedges for added brightness.

This simple and elegant dish is loaded with fresh flavors and takes under 30 minutes to prepare! Perfect for a healthy, satisfying meal.

8.   Vegetable Pad Thai with Almond Butter Sauce

Ingredients:

For the Pad Thai:

- 8 ounces rice noodles (thin or wide)

- 1 tablespoon sesame oil (or any neutral oil)

- 1 medium carrot, julienned or shredded

- 1 red bell pepper, thinly sliced

- 1 cup broccoli florets

- 2 cups bean sprouts

- 3 green onions, sliced

- 1/4 cup fresh cilantro, chopped (optional)

- 1/4 cup crushed peanuts, for garnish

- Lime wedges, for serving

For the Almond Butter Sauce:

- 1/4 cup almond butter (creamy and unsweetened)

- 3 tablespoons soy sauce (or tamari for gluten-free)

- 1 tablespoon rice vinegar

- 1 tablespoon lime juice

- 1 tablespoon maple syrup (or honey)

- 1 teaspoon sesame oil

- 1-2 tablespoons warm water (to thin, as needed)

- 1/2 teaspoon red pepper flakes (optional, for heat)

Instructions:

1. Prepare the Noodles:

    1. Cook the rice noodles according to package instructions. Drain and rinse with cold water to prevent sticking. Set aside.

2. Make the Almond Butter Sauce:

    1. In a small bowl, whisk together almond butter, soy sauce, rice vinegar, lime juice, maple syrup, sesame oil, and red pepper flakes (if using).

    2. Add warm water 1 tablespoon at a time, whisking until the sauce reaches a pourable consistency. Set aside.

3. Cook the Vegetables:

    1. Heat sesame oil in a large skillet or wok over medium-high heat.

    2. Add the carrot, bell pepper, and broccoli. Stir-fry for 4-5 minutes, or until the vegetables are tender-crisp.

4. Combine:

1.   Add the cooked rice noodles and bean sprouts to the skillet. Pour the almond butter sauce over the top and toss to coat everything evenly.

2.   Cook for 1-2 minutes until heated through.

5. Serve:

1.   Divide the Pad Thai into bowls or plates. Garnish with green onions, cilantro, crushed peanuts, and lime wedges.

2.   Serve warm and enjoy!

This Vegetable Pad Thai is a healthy, vibrant twist on the classic dish, with the almond butter sauce providing a creamy and flavorful touch! Perfect for a quick weeknight dinner.

9.   Rosemary-Roasted Sweet Potato and Carrot Medley

Ingredients:

- 2 medium sweet potatoes, peeled and cut into 1-inch cubes

- 4 large carrots, peeled and sliced into thick rounds

- 2 tablespoons olive oil

- 2 teaspoons fresh rosemary, chopped (or 1 teaspoon dried rosemary)

- 1 teaspoon garlic powder

- 1/2 teaspoon paprika

- Salt and pepper, to taste

- 1 tablespoon honey or maple syrup (optional, for sweetness)

Instructions:

1. Preheat the Oven:

1. Preheat your oven to 400°F (200°C). Line a large baking sheet with parchment paper or lightly grease it.

2. Prepare the Vegetables:

1. In a large bowl, toss the sweet potatoes and carrots with olive oil, rosemary, garlic powder, paprika, salt, and pepper.

2. If using, drizzle with honey or maple syrup and toss again to coat evenly.

3. Roast:

1. Spread the vegetables in a single layer on the prepared baking sheet.

2. Roast for 25-30 minutes, stirring halfway through, until the vegetables are tender and lightly caramelized.

4. Serve:

1. Transfer to a serving dish and garnish with additional fresh rosemary, if desired.

2. Serve warm as a side dish or enjoy on its own!

This Rosemary-Roasted Sweet Potato and Carrot Medley is a simple, flavorful dish that's perfect for any occasion. The rosemary and touch of sweetness complement the natural flavors of the vegetables beautifully!

10. Slow-Cooked Turmeric and Ginger Chicken Stew

Ingredients:

*   1 1/2 pounds boneless, skinless chicken thighs, cut into large chunks

*   1 tablespoon olive oil

*   1 medium onion, finely chopped

*   3 garlic cloves, minced

*   1 tablespoon fresh ginger, grated (or 1 teaspoon ground ginger)

*   1 teaspoon ground turmeric

*   1 teaspoon ground cumin

*   1/2 teaspoon ground coriander

*   1/2 teaspoon smoked paprika

*   1/4 teaspoon cayenne pepper (optional, for heat)

*   2 medium carrots, sliced

*   1 medium sweet potato, peeled and diced

*   1 (14-ounce) can diced tomatoes

*   2 cups chicken broth

*   1 (14-ounce) can coconut milk

*   1/2 teaspoon salt, or to taste

- 1/4 teaspoon black pepper, or to taste

- Juice of 1/2 lemon

- Fresh cilantro, for garnish

Instructions:

1. Sear the Chicken:

    1. Heat olive oil in a skillet over medium-high heat. Add the chicken pieces and sear for 2-3 minutes on each side, until lightly browned (no need to cook through). Transfer to a slow cooker.

2. Sauté Aromatics:

    1. In the same skillet, sauté the onion for 3-4 minutes until softened.

    2. Add the garlic, ginger, turmeric, cumin, coriander, paprika, and cayenne (if using). Stir and cook for 1 minute until fragrant.

3. Assemble the Stew:

    1. Transfer the onion and spice mixture to the slow cooker.

    2. Add the carrots, sweet potato, diced tomatoes, chicken broth, and coconut milk. Stir to combine.

    3. Season with salt and pepper.

4. Cook:

    1. Cover and cook on low for 6-7 hours or high for 3-4 hours, until the chicken is tender and the vegetables are soft.

5. Finish and Serve:

    1. Stir in the lemon juice before serving for a bright, fresh flavor.

    2. Ladle the stew into bowls and garnish with fresh cilantro.

This Slow-Cooked Turmeric and Ginger Chicken Stew is hearty, aromatic, and packed with anti-inflammatory spices. Perfect for a comforting, nutritious meal!

Chapter 5

Healing Snacks and Sides (10 Recipes)

1. Sweet Potato Fries with Turmeric and Black Pepper

These baked sweet potato fries are a flavorful and anti-inflammatory twist on a classic favorite. Sweet potatoes are rich in beta-carotene and fiber, while turmeric and black pepper combine to boost anti-inflammatory benefits. A crispy, golden exterior and warm, spicy flavor make this dish a perfect side or snack.

Ingredients (Serves 4)

- 2 large sweet potatoes, peeled and cut into fries

- 2 tbsp olive oil

- 1 tsp turmeric powder

- 1/2 tsp garlic powder

- 1/4 tsp smoked paprika (optional, for a smoky flavor)

- 1/2 tsp black pepper, freshly ground

- 1/4 tsp sea salt, or to taste

Optional Dipping Sauce:

- 1/4 cup plain Greek yogurt (or dairy-free alternative)

- 1 tsp lemon juice

- 1/2 tsp honey

- Pinch of turmeric for extra flavor

Instructions

1. Preheat the Oven:

- Preheat your oven to 425°F (220°C). Line a baking sheet with parchment paper or lightly grease it with olive oil.

2. Prepare the Sweet Potato Fries:

- In a large bowl, toss the sweet potato fries with olive oil, ensuring each piece is lightly coated.

- In a small bowl, mix the turmeric, garlic powder, smoked paprika (if using), black pepper, and salt. Sprinkle the spice mixture over the fries and toss to coat evenly.

3. Bake the Fries:

- Spread the sweet potato fries in a single layer on the prepared baking sheet. Avoid overcrowding to ensure even crisping.

- Bake for 25-30 minutes, flipping the fries halfway through, until they are golden brown and crispy on the edges.

4. Make the Dipping Sauce (Optional):

- In a small bowl, whisk together Greek yogurt, lemon juice, honey, and a pinch of turmeric. Adjust seasoning to taste.

5. Serve:

- Remove the fries from the oven and allow them to cool slightly. Serve warm with the optional dipping sauce or enjoy on their own.

2. Guacamole with Flaxseed Crackers

This classic guacamole recipe is paired with crunchy flaxseed crackers for a nutrient-packed, anti-inflammatory snack. Avocados are rich in healthy fats and antioxidants, while flaxseeds provide omega-3 fatty acids and fiber, making this duo perfect for boosting overall health.

Ingredients

For the Guacamole:

- 2 ripe avocados

- 1 small tomato, diced

- 1/4 red onion, finely chopped

- 1 clove garlic, minced

- 1 tbsp fresh lime juice

- 1/4 tsp ground cumin (optional)

- 1/4 tsp sea salt, or to taste

- 1 tbsp fresh cilantro, chopped (optional)

- 1/2 jalapeño, finely chopped (optional, for heat)

For the Flaxseed Crackers:

- 1 cup ground flaxseeds

- 1/4 cup whole flaxseeds

- 1/2 tsp garlic powder

- 1/2 tsp onion powder

- 1/4 tsp sea salt

- 1/3 cup water, plus more if needed

Instructions

Step 1: Make the Flaxseed Crackers

1.   Preheat your oven to 350°F (175°C). Line a baking sheet with parchment paper.

2.   In a medium bowl, combine ground flaxseeds, whole flaxseeds, garlic powder, onion powder, and sea salt.

3.   Gradually add water, mixing until the mixture forms a thick dough. Add a little more water if the dough is too dry.

4.   Place the dough on the parchment-lined baking sheet. Cover with another sheet of parchment paper and roll out the dough until it is about 1/8 inch thick.

5.   Remove the top parchment sheet and score the dough into cracker-sized pieces using a knife or pizza cutter.

6.   Bake for 15-20 minutes, or until crispy and golden brown. Let cool completely before breaking into pieces.

Step 2: Make the Guacamole

1.   Cut the avocados in half, remove the pit, and scoop the flesh into a bowl. Mash with a fork to your desired consistency (chunky or smooth).

2.   Add diced tomato, chopped onion, minced garlic, lime juice, cumin, sea salt, and cilantro. Mix well to combine.

3.   Taste and adjust seasoning as needed. If you like a bit of heat, mix in finely chopped jalapeño.

Step 3: Serve

• Serve the guacamole in a bowl alongside the flaxseed crackers. Enjoy as a snack, appetizer, or even a light meal!

Why It's Anti-Inflammatory

• Avocado: Rich in monounsaturated fats, vitamin E, and antioxidants, avocados help reduce inflammation and promote heart and brain health.

• Flaxseeds: Contain alpha-linolenic acid (ALA), an omega-3 fatty acid with anti-inflammatory properties, as well as lignans that support gut health.

• Lime Juice: High in vitamin C, which helps combat oxidative stress and inflammation.

• Garlic: A natural anti-inflammatory, garlic supports immune function and has antimicrobial benefits.

3.   Roasted Brussels Sprouts with Balsamic Glaze

This simple yet flavorful side dish features crispy roasted Brussels sprouts drizzled with a tangy-sweet balsamic glaze. Brussels sprouts are nutrient-dense and packed with anti-inflammatory properties, making this dish a perfect addition to any meal.

Ingredients (Serves 4)

• 1 lb (450 g) Brussels sprouts, trimmed and halved

• 2 tbsp olive oil

• 1/4 tsp sea salt, or to taste

- 1/4 tsp black pepper, freshly ground

- 1/4 cup balsamic vinegar

- 1 tbsp honey (or maple syrup for a vegan option)

- 1 tbsp toasted slivered almonds or pumpkin seeds (optional, for garnish)

Instructions

1. Preheat the Oven:

- Preheat your oven to 400°F (200°C) and line a baking sheet with parchment paper.

2. Prepare the Brussels Sprouts:

- In a large bowl, toss the halved Brussels sprouts with olive oil, sea salt, and black pepper until evenly coated.

3. Roast:

- Spread the Brussels sprouts in a single layer on the prepared baking sheet, cut side down for optimal caramelization.

- Roast for 20-25 minutes, flipping halfway through, until the edges are crispy and golden brown.

4. Make the Balsamic Glaze:

- While the Brussels sprouts roast, combine the balsamic vinegar and honey (or maple syrup) in a small saucepan over medium heat.

- Simmer gently, stirring occasionally, until the mixture thickens slightly and reduces by half (about 5-7 minutes). Remove from heat.

5. Assemble the Dish:

• Once the Brussels sprouts are roasted, transfer them to a serving bowl or platter. Drizzle the balsamic glaze over the top.

• Garnish with toasted slivered almonds or pumpkin seeds for added crunch, if desired.

6. Serve:

• Serve warm as a side dish or light appetizer.

4. Golden Milk Energy Bites (Turmeric, Dates, and Nuts)

These Golden Milk Energy Bites are a convenient, no-bake snack inspired by the warming flavors of turmeric-infused golden milk. Packed with anti-inflammatory spices, natural sweetness from dates, and healthy fats from nuts, these bites are perfect for an energy boost or a guilt-free treat.

Ingredients (Makes 12-15 bites)

• 1 cup medjool dates, pitted (about 10-12 dates)

• 1/2 cup raw almonds

• 1/2 cup raw cashews

• 1/4 cup shredded unsweetened coconut

• 1 tbsp ground turmeric

• 1/2 tsp ground cinnamon

• 1/4 tsp ground ginger

- 1/4 tsp black pepper (enhances turmeric's absorption)

- 1 tsp vanilla extract

- 1-2 tsp coconut oil, melted (if needed for consistency)

- Optional garnish: Additional shredded coconut for rolling

Instructions

1.   Prepare the Dates:

- Soak the pitted dates in warm water for 5-10 minutes if they're not soft. Drain well before use.

2.   Blend the Ingredients:

- In a food processor, combine the dates, almonds, cashews, shredded coconut, turmeric, cinnamon, ginger, black pepper, and vanilla extract.

- Process until the mixture comes together into a sticky, dough-like consistency. If the mixture is too dry, add 1-2 teaspoons of melted coconut oil and pulse again.

3.   Form the Energy Bites:

- Scoop out about 1 tablespoon of the mixture at a time and roll it between your palms to form small balls.

- Optional: Roll each ball in shredded coconut for added texture and visual appeal.

4.   Chill and Store:

- Place the energy bites on a parchment-lined tray and refrigerate for 30 minutes to firm up.

- Store in an airtight container in the refrigerator for up to 2 weeks or in the freezer for up to 3 months.

5.   Hummus Trio: Beet, Turmeric, and Classic Chickpea

This vibrant hummus trio combines three delicious and nutrient-packed varieties: Beet Hummus, Turmeric Hummus, and Classic Chickpea Hummus. Each version is rich in anti-inflammatory ingredients and perfect for snacking, dipping, or spreading.

Base Ingredients

For each hummus:

- 1 1/2 cups cooked chickpeas (or 1 can, drained and rinsed)

- 1/4 cup tahini

- 2 tbsp olive oil

- 2 tbsp fresh lemon juice

- 1 small garlic clove, minced

- 1/4 tsp sea salt (or to taste)

- 2-4 tbsp water (adjust for desired consistency)

Beet Hummus Ingredients

- 1/2 cup cooked beet, chopped

- 1/4 tsp ground cumin

- 1/4 tsp paprika

Turmeric Hummus Ingredients

- 1/2 tsp ground turmeric

- 1/4 tsp ground ginger

- 1/8 tsp black pepper (enhances turmeric absorption)

Classic Chickpea Hummus Ingredients

- 1/4 tsp ground cumin

- Optional garnish: Paprika and chopped parsley

Instructions

1. Prepare the Base:

- In a food processor, combine the chickpeas, tahini, olive oil, lemon juice, garlic, and sea salt. Blend until smooth.

- Add water, 1 tablespoon at a time, to reach your desired consistency.

2. Create Each Flavor:

- Beet Hummus: Add the chopped beet, cumin, and paprika to the base. Blend until smooth and vibrant pink.

- Turmeric Hummus: Add the turmeric, ginger, and black pepper to the base. Blend until smooth and golden yellow.

- Classic Hummus: Add the cumin to the base and blend until smooth.

3. Taste and Adjust:

- Adjust salt, lemon juice, or spices to your liking for each hummus flavor.

4. Serve and Garnish:

- Transfer each hummus to a separate bowl. Garnish the Beet Hummus with a drizzle of olive oil and sesame seeds, the Turmeric Hummus with a sprinkle of turmeric and black sesame seeds, and the Classic Hummus with paprika and parsley.

5.   Store:

•   Store in airtight containers in the refrigerator for up to 5 days.

Why It's Anti-Inflammatory

•   Beets: High in betalains, which reduce inflammation and support detoxification.

•   Turmeric and Black Pepper: Boost anti-inflammatory properties through curcumin and piperine.

•   Chickpeas and Olive Oil: Provide fiber, healthy fats, and antioxidants that combat inflammation.

6.   Spiced Pumpkin Seeds

These Spiced Pumpkin Seeds are a crunchy, flavorful snack rich in anti-inflammatory nutrients like magnesium, zinc, and omega-3 fatty acids. They're quick to prepare and perfect for munching, topping salads, or garnishing soups.

Ingredients

•   1 cup raw pumpkin seeds (pepitas)

•   1 tbsp olive oil or coconut oil

•   1/2 tsp ground turmeric

•   1/2 tsp smoked paprika

•   1/4 tsp ground cumin

- 1/4 tsp ground cinnamon

- 1/4 tsp garlic powder

- 1/4 tsp sea salt

- 1/8 tsp black pepper (optional, for turmeric absorption)

Instructions

1. Preheat the Oven:

- Preheat your oven to 325°F (160°C) and line a baking sheet with parchment paper.

2. Mix the Spices:

- In a small bowl, combine turmeric, smoked paprika, cumin, cinnamon, garlic powder, salt, and black pepper (if using).

3. Prepare the Pumpkin Seeds:

- In a mixing bowl, toss the pumpkin seeds with olive oil, ensuring they are evenly coated.

- Add the spice mixture to the seeds and toss well to coat evenly.

4. Bake:

- Spread the seasoned pumpkin seeds in a single layer on the prepared baking sheet.

- Bake for 12-15 minutes, stirring halfway through, until they are golden and crisp.

5. Cool and Store:

- Let the seeds cool completely on the baking sheet.

- Store in an airtight container at room temperature for up to 2 weeks.

7. Roasted Cauliflower with Cumin and Lemon

This Roasted Cauliflower with Cumin and Lemon is a simple, nutrient-packed side dish bursting with flavor. Cauliflower's natural nuttiness pairs perfectly with the earthy warmth of cumin and the bright tang of lemon, making it a delicious addition to any anti-inflammatory meal.

Ingredients

- 1 medium cauliflower, cut into florets

- 2 tbsp olive oil

- 1 tsp ground cumin

- 1/2 tsp turmeric powder

- 1/4 tsp smoked paprika

- 1/2 tsp sea salt (or to taste)

- 1/4 tsp black pepper

- 1 lemon (zest and juice)

- Fresh parsley, chopped (optional, for garnish)

Instructions

1. Preheat the Oven:

- Preheat your oven to 400°F (200°C) and line a baking sheet with parchment paper.

2. Season the Cauliflower:

- In a large mixing bowl, toss the cauliflower florets with olive oil.

• Add cumin, turmeric, smoked paprika, salt, and black pepper, and mix until the florets are evenly coated.

3.   Roast the Cauliflower:

• Spread the seasoned cauliflower in a single layer on the prepared baking sheet.

• Roast for 25-30 minutes, stirring halfway through, until the cauliflower is golden and tender.

4.   Add Lemon:

• Remove the cauliflower from the oven and immediately drizzle with lemon juice and sprinkle with lemon zest. Toss gently to combine.

5.   Garnish and Serve:

• Transfer the roasted cauliflower to a serving dish and garnish with fresh parsley, if desired.

Why It's Anti-Inflammatory

• Cauliflower: A cruciferous vegetable rich in antioxidants and compounds like sulforaphane, which fight inflammation.

• Turmeric: Contains curcumin, a powerful anti-inflammatory compound.

• Lemon: High in vitamin C, which helps neutralize free radicals and reduce oxidative stress.

• Cumin: Supports digestion and has antioxidant properties.

8. Cucumber Slices with Herbed Greek Yogurt Dip

This refreshing and flavorful snack combines hydrating cucumber slices with a creamy, herbed Greek yogurt dip. Packed with anti-inflammatory ingredients, it's perfect as an appetizer, side dish, or healthy snack.

Ingredients

For the Cucumber Slices:

- 1 large cucumber, sliced into thin rounds

- Pinch of sea salt (optional)

For the Herbed Greek Yogurt Dip:

- 1 cup plain Greek yogurt (unsweetened, full-fat or low-fat)

- 1 tbsp olive oil

- 1 tbsp lemon juice (freshly squeezed)

- 1 clove garlic, finely minced

- 1 tbsp fresh dill, chopped

- 1 tbsp fresh parsley, chopped

- 1/2 tsp ground cumin

- 1/4 tsp turmeric (optional for added anti-inflammatory benefits)

- 1/4 tsp sea salt (or to taste)

- 1/4 tsp black pepper

Instructions

1. Prepare the Dip:

•	In a mixing bowl, combine the Greek yogurt, olive oil, lemon juice, and minced garlic.

•	Stir in the chopped dill, parsley, cumin, turmeric (if using), salt, and pepper. Mix well until all the ingredients are fully incorporated.

2.	Chill the Dip:

•	Cover the bowl and refrigerate for at least 15 minutes to allow the flavors to meld together.

3.	Prepare the Cucumber:

•	Slice the cucumber into thin rounds. Sprinkle with a pinch of sea salt if desired.

4.	Serve:

•	Arrange the cucumber slices on a plate and serve alongside the herbed Greek yogurt dip.

Why It's Anti-Inflammatory

•	Cucumber: Hydrating and rich in antioxidants like beta-carotene, which helps reduce inflammation.

•	Greek Yogurt: Contains probiotics that promote gut health and reduce inflammation.

•	Olive Oil: A source of healthy fats and anti-inflammatory compounds like oleocanthal.

•	Herbs (Dill and Parsley): High in antioxidants and phytonutrients that combat oxidative stress.

•	Turmeric and Cumin: Powerful spices with proven anti-inflammatory and digestive benefits.

9. Carrot and Ginger Slaw with Sesame Seeds

This vibrant Carrot and Ginger Slaw is a refreshing, crunchy dish packed with anti-inflammatory ingredients like fresh ginger, carrots, and sesame seeds. It's perfect as a side dish, salad topper, or a light snack.

Ingredients

- 3 cups carrots, shredded or julienned

- 1/4 cup red cabbage, thinly sliced (optional for extra color and nutrients)

- 1 tbsp fresh ginger, finely grated

- 2 tbsp sesame seeds (toasted, if desired)

- 2 green onions, thinly sliced

- 1 tbsp fresh cilantro, chopped (optional)

For the Dressing:

- 2 tbsp olive oil or sesame oil

- 1 tbsp rice vinegar or apple cider vinegar

- 1 tbsp fresh lime juice

- 1 tsp honey or maple syrup (optional, for a hint of sweetness)

- 1/2 tsp sea salt

- 1/4 tsp black pepper

Instructions

1. Prepare the Vegetables:

•   In a large mixing bowl, combine the shredded carrots, red cabbage (if using), green onions, and cilantro.

2.   Make the Dressing:

•   In a small bowl, whisk together olive oil (or sesame oil), rice vinegar, lime juice, grated ginger, honey (if using), sea salt, and black pepper.

3.   Combine:

•   Pour the dressing over the vegetables and toss until everything is evenly coated.

4.   Add Sesame Seeds:

•   Sprinkle the sesame seeds over the slaw and gently mix.

5.   Chill and Serve:

•   Let the slaw sit for 10-15 minutes to allow the flavors to meld, then serve immediately.

Why It's Anti-Inflammatory

•   Carrots: Rich in beta-carotene and antioxidants that combat inflammation.

•   Ginger: Contains gingerol, a potent anti-inflammatory compound.

•   Sesame Seeds: A source of magnesium, healthy fats, and lignans that reduce inflammation.

•   Olive Oil: Provides anti-inflammatory oleocanthal.

10. Avocado and Cucumber Summer Rolls with Almond Dipping Sauce

These refreshing summer rolls are packed with hydrating cucumber, creamy avocado, and fresh herbs, making them a perfect light and anti-inflammatory meal. Paired with a flavorful almond dipping sauce, they're both satisfying and nutrient-rich.

Ingredients

For the Summer Rolls:

- 8 rice paper wrappers

- 1 avocado, thinly sliced

- 1/2 cucumber, julienned

- 1 medium carrot, julienned

- 1/2 cup red bell pepper, julienned

- 1/4 cup fresh cilantro

- 1/4 cup fresh mint leaves

- 1/4 cup fresh basil leaves

- Optional: 1/2 cup cooked rice noodles or julienned zucchini noodles

For the Almond Dipping Sauce:

- 1/4 cup almond butter (unsweetened)

- 2 tbsp tamari or low-sodium soy sauce

- 1 tbsp rice vinegar or apple cider vinegar

- 1 tbsp fresh lime juice

- 1 tsp honey or maple syrup

- 1/2 tsp fresh ginger, grated

- 2-3 tbsp water (to adjust consistency)

Instructions

1. Prepare the Almond Dipping Sauce:

- In a small bowl, whisk together almond butter, tamari, rice vinegar, lime juice, honey, and grated ginger.

- Add water a tablespoon at a time until the sauce reaches your desired consistency. Set aside.

2. Prepare the Filling:

- Arrange all the filling ingredients (avocado, cucumber, carrot, red bell pepper, and fresh herbs) on a platter for easy assembly.

3. Soften the Rice Paper Wrappers:

- Fill a large, shallow dish with warm water.

- Working one at a time, dip a rice paper wrapper into the water for 10-15 seconds until soft but not overly pliable. Remove and place on a clean, damp surface.

4. Assemble the Summer Rolls:

- Place a few slices of avocado, cucumber, carrot, red bell pepper, and a small handful of herbs in the center of the wrapper. Add noodles if using.

• Fold the sides of the wrapper inward, then tightly roll it up from the bottom like a burrito. Repeat with the remaining wrappers and fillings.

5. Serve:

• Slice the summer rolls in half and serve with the almond dipping sauce on the side.

Why It's Anti-Inflammatory

• Avocado: Packed with healthy fats and antioxidants that reduce inflammation.

• Cucumber: Hydrating and rich in compounds that combat oxidative stress.

• Fresh Herbs: Cilantro, mint, and basil are loaded with phytonutrients and anti-inflammatory properties.

• Almond Butter: A source of vitamin E and healthy fats that promote overall cellular health.

• Ginger: Known for its potent anti-inflammatory effects.

Chapter 6

Anti-Inflammatory Desserts and Drinks (10 Recipes)

1. Dark Chocolate Avocado Mousse

This indulgent yet healthy dessert combines the rich taste of dark chocolate with the creamy texture of avocado, creating a decadent mousse that's full of healthy fats, antioxidants, and anti-inflammatory benefits. Perfect for satisfying your sweet tooth without the guilt!

Ingredients

- 2 ripe avocados, peeled and pitted

- 1/4 cup unsweetened cocoa powder

- 1/4 cup dark chocolate chips (70% cocoa or higher)

- 2-3 tbsp maple syrup (or honey, to taste)

- 1 tsp vanilla extract

- Pinch of sea salt

- 2 tbsp almond milk (or any plant-based milk)

- Optional toppings: fresh berries, chopped nuts, or a sprinkle of cacao nibs

Instructions

1.   Melt the Chocolate:

•   Place the dark chocolate chips in a heatproof bowl. Melt them using a double boiler method (place the bowl over simmering water) or microwave in 20-second intervals, stirring in between until fully melted.

2.   Blend the Ingredients:

•   In a food processor or blender, combine the ripe avocados, melted chocolate, cocoa powder, maple syrup, vanilla extract, and a pinch of sea salt.

•   Blend until smooth and creamy. If the mousse is too thick, add almond milk one tablespoon at a time until you reach your desired consistency.

3.   Chill:

•   Transfer the mousse into serving bowls or glasses and refrigerate for at least 1 hour to allow the flavors to meld and the mousse to set.

4.   Serve:

•   Before serving, top with fresh berries, chopped nuts, or cacao nibs for an added texture and flavor boost.

Why It's Anti-Inflammatory

•   Avocado: Rich in healthy monounsaturated fats, antioxidants, and anti-inflammatory compounds that help reduce oxidative stress.

•   Dark Chocolate: Contains flavonoids, especially epicatechin, which have been shown to lower inflammation and protect heart health.

•   Cocoa: Packed with polyphenols, particularly flavonoids, that fight inflammation and support overall health.

•   Almond Milk: A dairy-free alternative that provides a smooth texture and contains anti-inflammatory omega-3s (depending on the brand).

2.   Berry and Coconut Yogurt Parfait

This refreshing and nutritious parfait layers antioxidant-rich berries with creamy coconut yogurt and crunchy granola, making it a delicious and anti-inflammatory breakfast or snack. The combination of fiber, healthy fats, and probiotics provides a perfect balance for your gut health and overall well-being.

Ingredients

•   1 cup coconut yogurt (unsweetened, dairy-free)

•   1/2 cup fresh mixed berries (blueberries, raspberries, strawberries, blackberries)

•   2 tbsp chia seeds

•   1 tbsp flaxseeds (optional)

•   1/4 cup granola (preferably low-sugar and whole-grain)

•   1 tbsp unsweetened shredded coconut

•   1-2 tsp honey or maple syrup (optional, depending on sweetness preference)

•   Fresh mint leaves (for garnish)

Instructions

1.   Prepare the Yogurt Base:

•   In a small bowl, mix the coconut yogurt with chia seeds, flaxseeds (if using), and honey or maple syrup (if desired). Stir well to combine, and let it sit for about 5-10 minutes to allow the chia seeds to absorb the liquid and thicken the mixture.

2.   Assemble the Parfait:

•   In serving glasses or bowls, layer the coconut yogurt mixture at the bottom.

•   Add a layer of mixed berries, followed by a layer of granola. Repeat the layers until you reach the top of the glass.

3.   Top with Garnishes:

•   Finish with a sprinkle of shredded coconut, a few extra berries, and a fresh mint leaf for a touch of color and freshness.

4.   Chill (Optional):

•   For a more refreshing treat, refrigerate the parfaits for 20-30 minutes before serving to allow the flavors to meld together.

Why It's Anti-Inflammatory

•   Berries: Rich in antioxidants like anthocyanins and flavonoids, berries help reduce oxidative stress and inflammation, protecting the body from chronic diseases.

•   Coconut Yogurt: A dairy-free probiotic option that supports gut health and reduces inflammation. It's also rich in healthy fats, which help decrease inflammation at the cellular level.

•   Chia Seeds: Packed with omega-3 fatty acids, fiber, and antioxidants, chia seeds support heart health and help reduce systemic inflammation.

• Flaxseeds: Rich in lignans and omega-3s, flaxseeds are known for their ability to reduce inflammation and promote overall well-being.

• Granola: Opting for whole-grain granola adds fiber, which helps stabilize blood sugar levels and fight inflammation.

3. Cinnamon-Baked Apples with Walnuts

This warm, comforting dessert is a perfect way to enjoy anti-inflammatory ingredients while satisfying your sweet tooth. The combination of cinnamon, apples, and walnuts offers a delicious mix of antioxidants, fiber, and healthy fats that can help reduce inflammation and promote overall health.

Ingredients

• 4 medium apples (choose a firm variety like Granny Smith, Honeycrisp, or Gala)

• 1/4 cup walnuts, chopped

• 1 tbsp cinnamon

• 1 tbsp honey or maple syrup (optional)

• 1 tbsp coconut oil (or butter)

• 1/2 tsp vanilla extract

• 1/4 tsp ground ginger (optional)

• 1/4 tsp ground nutmeg (optional)

• Pinch of sea salt

Instructions

1. Preheat the Oven:

• Preheat your oven to 350°F (175°C).

2. Prepare the Apples:

• Core the apples, leaving the bottom intact to form a hollow center for the filling. You can use an apple corer or carefully cut a cone-shaped core out of the apples with a knife.

• Place the apples in a baking dish that's just large enough to hold them upright.

3. Make the Filling:

• In a small bowl, combine the chopped walnuts, cinnamon, honey (or maple syrup), vanilla extract, ginger, nutmeg, and a pinch of sea salt. Stir to combine.

4. Stuff the Apples:

• Fill the hollowed centers of each apple with the walnut mixture, packing it tightly.

• Top each apple with a small dollop of coconut oil (or butter) to help with the baking process.

5. Bake the Apples:

• Cover the baking dish with aluminum foil and bake for about 30-40 minutes, or until the apples are tender but not mushy. You can check the tenderness by poking the apples with a fork.

6. Serve:

• Once baked, remove the apples from the oven and allow them to cool slightly before serving. They can be enjoyed as is or topped with a drizzle of extra honey or a sprinkle of cinnamon if desired.

4. Chilled Matcha Latte with Almond Milk

This refreshing iced matcha latte is a soothing and energizing drink that combines the antioxidant-rich power of matcha with the creamy goodness of almond milk. The combination of green tea's natural caffeine and almond milk's healthy fats makes it a perfect anti-inflammatory beverage to enjoy any time of the day.

Ingredients

- 1 tsp matcha powder (high-quality, organic)

- 1 cup unsweetened almond milk

- 1-2 tsp honey or maple syrup (optional, depending on sweetness preference)

- 1/2 tsp vanilla extract

- 1/4 tsp ground cinnamon (optional, for extra flavor)

- Ice cubes (as needed)

Instructions

1. Prepare the Matcha:

- In a small bowl, sift the matcha powder to remove any clumps.

- Add about 2 tablespoons of hot water (not boiling, about 175°F or 80°C) to the matcha powder and whisk it using a bamboo whisk or small electric frother until the matcha is fully dissolved and forms a smooth paste.

2. Mix the Latte:

• In a separate cup or shaker, combine the unsweetened almond milk, vanilla extract, and honey or maple syrup.

• Add the matcha paste to the milk mixture and stir or shake well to combine.

3. Serve:

• Fill a glass with ice cubes, then pour the matcha latte over the ice.

• Optionally, sprinkle a dash of ground cinnamon on top for added flavor.

4. Enjoy:

• Stir to combine and enjoy your chilled, refreshing matcha latte!

5. Hibiscus and Ginger Iced Tea

This vibrant and refreshing iced tea combines the tart, floral notes of hibiscus with the spicy warmth of ginger. Both ingredients are known for their powerful anti-inflammatory and antioxidant properties, making this a perfect drink to cool off and support your health simultaneously.

Ingredients

• 2 tbsp dried hibiscus flowers (or 2 hibiscus tea bags)

• 1-inch piece of fresh ginger, peeled and sliced

• 1-2 tsp honey or maple syrup (optional, adjust to sweetness preference)

- 4 cups water

- Ice cubes

- 1-2 slices of lemon (optional, for garnish)

Instructions

1. Boil the Water:

- In a medium saucepan, bring 4 cups of water to a boil.

2. Prepare the Tea:

- Once the water has boiled, remove it from the heat and add the dried hibiscus flowers and sliced ginger to the pot.

- Cover and steep the tea for about 10-15 minutes, depending on how strong you prefer the flavor. The longer it steeps, the more robust the flavors will be.

3. Sweeten the Tea:

- After steeping, strain the tea into a pitcher, discarding the hibiscus flowers and ginger slices.

- Stir in honey or maple syrup while the tea is still warm, allowing it to dissolve fully.

4. Cool the Tea:

- Let the tea cool to room temperature, then transfer it to the refrigerator and chill for at least 1 hour.

5. Serve:

- Fill a glass with ice cubes and pour the chilled tea over the ice.

- Garnish with a slice of lemon for extra freshness and flavor.

6. Enjoy:

• Stir well and enjoy the tart, refreshing flavor of your hibiscus and ginger iced tea!

6. Dairy-Free Turmeric Latte

Also known as "Golden Milk," this dairy-free turmeric latte is a soothing, vibrant beverage with powerful anti-inflammatory properties. The combination of turmeric, coconut milk, and other spices helps support joint health, reduce inflammation, and improve digestion. Enjoy this warm, creamy drink anytime you need a calming, healthy treat.

Ingredients

• 1 cup coconut milk (or other non-dairy milk like almond or oat milk)

• 1 tsp ground turmeric

• 1/2 tsp ground ginger

• 1/4 tsp ground cinnamon

• 1/4 tsp black pepper (to enhance the absorption of turmeric)

• 1 tsp honey or maple syrup (optional, adjust to sweetness preference)

• 1/2 tsp vanilla extract (optional)

• Pinch of sea salt (optional)

Instructions

1. Heat the Milk:

• In a small saucepan, heat the coconut milk over medium heat until it's warm but not boiling. Stir occasionally to prevent it from scorching.

2.   Add the Spices:

•   Add the turmeric, ginger, cinnamon, black pepper, and vanilla extract (if using) to the warm milk. Whisk the ingredients together until they are well combined.

3.   Sweeten the Latte:

•   Stir in honey or maple syrup to taste. You can adjust the sweetness based on your preference.

4.   Simmer:

•   Lower the heat and let the mixture simmer for 2-3 minutes, allowing the flavors to blend together.

5.   Serve:

•   Pour the turmeric latte into a mug. Optionally, sprinkle a pinch of cinnamon or ground turmeric on top for garnish.

6.   Enjoy:

•   Stir well and sip slowly, allowing the warm, soothing flavors to relax your body and mind.

7.   Chia Seed Mango Pudding

This vibrant, creamy chia seed pudding is made with fresh mango puree, providing a burst of tropical flavor. Chia seeds are packed with omega-3 fatty acids, fiber, and antioxidants, while the mango adds a rich source of vitamin C, making this a perfect anti-inflammatory dessert or snack.

Ingredients

- 1 cup coconut milk (or other non-dairy milk)

- 1/2 cup mango puree (about 1 ripe mango, peeled and blended)

- 3 tbsp chia seeds

- 1 tbsp maple syrup or honey (optional, adjust to sweetness preference)

- 1/2 tsp vanilla extract (optional)

- Pinch of sea salt (optional)

- Fresh mango slices for garnish (optional)

- Mint leaves for garnish (optional)

Instructions

1. Make the Mango Puree:

- If using fresh mango, peel and chop the mango into chunks. Blend it in a blender or food processor until smooth. You should have about 1/2 cup of mango puree.

2. Mix the Ingredients:

- In a mixing bowl or jar, combine the coconut milk, mango puree, maple syrup or honey (if using), vanilla extract, and a pinch of salt. Stir until well combined.

3. Add the Chia Seeds:

- Stir in the chia seeds, making sure they are evenly distributed throughout the mixture.

4. Let It Set:

• Cover the bowl or jar and refrigerate the mixture for at least 4 hours, or overnight. This allows the chia seeds to absorb the liquid and thicken the pudding.

5. Serve:

• Once the pudding has set, give it a good stir. Spoon it into serving bowls or jars.

6. Garnish and Enjoy:

• Garnish with fresh mango slices and mint leaves if desired. Serve chilled and enjoy!

8. Date and Almond Truffles with Cacao Powder

These Date and Almond Truffles are a perfect bite-sized treat for anyone looking for an anti-inflammatory snack that is rich in healthy fats, antioxidants, and natural sweetness. The combination of dates, almonds, and cacao powder provides a satisfying flavor, while also supporting inflammation reduction, digestive health, and overall wellness.

Ingredients

• 1 cup pitted dates (about 8-10 dates)

• 1/2 cup almonds (raw, unsalted)

• 2 tbsp raw cacao powder (or cocoa powder)

• 1 tsp vanilla extract

• 1/4 tsp ground cinnamon

- Pinch of sea salt

- 1 tbsp coconut oil (optional, for extra creaminess)

- Additional cacao powder or chopped almonds for rolling (optional)

Instructions

1. Prepare the Dates:

- If your dates are not soft, soak them in warm water for about 10 minutes to soften them up. Then drain and pat dry.

2. Blend the Ingredients:

- In a food processor, combine the dates, almonds, cacao powder, vanilla extract, cinnamon, and a pinch of salt. Blend until the mixture becomes sticky and begins to clump together. You may need to scrape down the sides of the processor bowl to ensure everything is well mixed.

3. Add Coconut Oil:

- If you want a creamier texture, add coconut oil to the mixture and pulse a few more times until fully combined.

4. Form the Truffles:

- Take small amounts of the mixture (about 1 tablespoon) and roll them into bite-sized balls using your hands.

5. Coat the Truffles:

- Roll the truffles in additional cacao powder or chopped almonds for an extra layer of flavor and texture.

6. Refrigerate:

• Place the truffles on a plate or tray and refrigerate them for at least 30 minutes to firm up.

7. Serve:

• Once chilled, serve and enjoy these sweet, nutrient-dense truffles!

9. Frozen Banana Bites with Dark Chocolate Drizzle

These Frozen Banana Bites with Dark Chocolate Drizzle are a simple, yet indulgent snack that combines the natural sweetness of bananas with the rich, antioxidant-packed benefits of dark chocolate. They are easy to make, perfectly satisfying, and great for anyone looking to enjoy an anti-inflammatory treat. Bananas provide potassium and fiber, while dark chocolate is known for its anti-inflammatory flavonoids.

Ingredients

• 2 ripe bananas

• 1/2 cup dark chocolate (70% or higher, chopped or in chips)

• 1 tbsp coconut oil (optional, for smoother chocolate drizzle)

• 1/4 tsp sea salt (optional, for sprinkling)

• Chopped nuts (such as almonds or walnuts, optional for topping)

• Shredded coconut (optional for topping)

Instructions

1.   Prepare the Bananas:

•   Peel the bananas and cut them into bite-sized slices, about 1-inch thick.

2.   Prepare the Chocolate Drizzle:

•   Place the dark chocolate in a microwave-safe bowl. If using coconut oil, add it to the bowl to help the chocolate melt smoothly.

•   Microwave the chocolate in 20-30 second intervals, stirring in between, until it is completely melted and smooth. Alternatively, melt the chocolate in a double boiler.

3.   Assemble the Banana Bites:

•   Lay the banana slices on a parchment-lined baking sheet. You can place them side by side, but make sure they don't touch each other.

4.   Drizzle the Chocolate:

•   Use a spoon or a small whisk to drizzle the melted dark chocolate over the banana slices. If desired, you can sprinkle a pinch of sea salt on top for a sweet-salty combination.

5.   Add Optional Toppings:

•   Sprinkle some chopped nuts or shredded coconut on top of the chocolate-covered banana bites for extra texture and flavor.

6.   Freeze:

•   Place the baking sheet with the banana bites in the freezer and let them freeze for at least 2 hours, or until firm.

7.   Serve and Enjoy:

•   Once frozen, the banana bites are ready to be enjoyed! Store any leftovers in an airtight container in the freezer.

10. Spiced Apple Cider with Cinnamon and Cloves

This Spiced Apple Cider with Cinnamon and Cloves is a warm, comforting beverage that is perfect for any time of year, especially when you're craving something cozy and anti-inflammatory. The combination of apples, cinnamon, and cloves not only provides a delicious, aromatic drink but also offers several health benefits. The spices are known to support digestion, reduce inflammation, and boost immunity.

Ingredients

- 4 cups apple cider (preferably fresh and unfiltered)

- 2 cinnamon sticks

- 4-6 whole cloves

- 1 star anise (optional, for additional flavor)

- 1/2 tsp ground ginger (or 1-2 slices of fresh ginger)

- 1 tbsp honey (or maple syrup for a vegan version, optional)

- 1/2 tsp vanilla extract (optional)

- Orange slices (for garnish, optional)

- Fresh cinnamon sticks (for garnish, optional)

Instructions

1. Combine the Ingredients:

•   In a medium saucepan, pour in the apple cider. Add the cinnamon sticks, cloves, star anise (if using), ground ginger (or fresh slices), and honey (or maple syrup).

2.   Heat the Cider:

•   Over medium heat, bring the cider to a simmer, stirring occasionally. Once it reaches a simmer, reduce the heat to low, and let the cider steep for about 10-15 minutes to allow the spices to infuse.

3.   Strain the Cider:

•   After simmering, remove the cider from the heat and strain it through a fine mesh strainer to remove the whole spices (cinnamon sticks, cloves, and ginger).

4.   Add Vanilla (Optional):

•   Stir in the vanilla extract, if desired, for an extra layer of flavor.

5.   Serve and Garnish:

•   Pour the spiced apple cider into mugs and garnish with fresh orange slices and additional cinnamon sticks, if desired.

6.   Enjoy:

•   Serve warm and enjoy the cozy, soothing flavors of the spiced cider.

Why It's Anti-Inflammatory

•   Apple Cider: Apple cider, particularly the unfiltered variety, contains antioxidants like polyphenols that help reduce oxidative stress and inflammation in the body. Apples themselves are high in fiber and vitamin C, which support digestion and immune function.

• Cinnamon: Cinnamon is a powerful anti-inflammatory spice. It contains compounds like cinnamaldehyde, which help reduce inflammation and can also support healthy blood sugar levels.

• Cloves: Cloves contain eugenol, a compound with potent anti-inflammatory and antioxidant properties. They have been shown to help reduce inflammation in the body and support digestive health.

• Ginger: Ginger is known for its ability to reduce inflammation and soothe the digestive tract. It contains bioactive compounds like gingerol that have anti-inflammatory effects.

• Honey: Honey, especially raw or manuka honey, has antibacterial and anti-inflammatory properties that can help support immune health and reduce inflammation.

This Spiced Apple Cider with Cinnamon and Cloves is the perfect anti-inflammatory drink to warm you up on a chilly day. The blend of spices not only provides comforting flavors but also offers health-boosting benefits. Would you like more ideas for warming, anti-inflammatory drinks or other cozy beverages?

Chapter 7

7-Day Anti-Inflammatory Meal Plan

Pre-planned meals combining recipes from all chapters.

This 7-Day Anti-Inflammatory Meal Plan combines recipes from various chapters, ensuring a balanced, nutrient-rich approach to eating that supports your health by reducing inflammation. Each day includes a variety of meals designed to nourish your body with anti-inflammatory ingredients like omega-3s, antioxidants, and fiber. These meals are designed to support digestion, boost immunity, and help manage chronic inflammation.

Day 1:

Breakfast:

- Golden Turmeric Overnight Oats

- Drink: Dairy-Free Turmeric Latte

Lunch:

- Quinoa Buddha Bowl with Roasted Veggies and Tahini Dressing

Snack:

- Spiced Pumpkin Seeds

Dinner:

- Lentil and Sweet Potato Stew

Day 2:

Breakfast:

- Sweet Potato and Kale Breakfast Hash

- Drink: Hibiscus and Ginger Iced Tea

Lunch:

- Wild-Caught Salmon Salad with Arugula and Pomegranate

Snack:

- Avocado and Cucumber Summer Rolls with Almond Dipping Sauce

Dinner:

- Zucchini Noodles with Pesto and Grilled Chicken

Day 3:

Breakfast:

- Blueberry Chia Pudding with Almond Milk

- Drink: Chilled Matcha Latte with Almond Milk

Lunch:

- Mediterranean Chickpea Salad with Lemon and Olive Oil

Snack:

- Carrot and Ginger Slaw with Sesame Seeds

Dinner:

- Spaghetti Squash with Tomato Basil Sauce

Day 4:

Breakfast:

- Spinach and Mushroom Omelette with Avocado

- Drink: Chia Seed Mango Pudding

Lunch:

- Lentil and Sweet Potato Stew

Snack:

- Roasted Brussels Sprouts with Balsamic Glaze

Dinner:

- Miso Soup with Tofu, Wakame, and Green Onions

Day 5:

Breakfast:

- Anti-Inflammatory Smoothie (Spinach, Pineapple, Ginger, Coconut Water)

- Drink: Date and Almond Truffles with Cacao Powder

Lunch:

- Grilled Shrimp Tacos with Mango Salsa

Snack:

- Cucumber Slices with Herbed Greek Yogurt Dip

Dinner:

- Turmeric-Spiced Cauliflower Soup

Day 6:

Breakfast:

- Matcha Coconut Pancakes with Berries

- Drink: Frozen Banana Bites with Dark Chocolate Drizzle

Lunch:

- Avocado and Hummus Wrap with Spinach and Cucumber

Snack:

- Hummus Trio (Beet, Turmeric, and Classic Chickpea)

Dinner:

- Grilled Shrimp Tacos with Mango Salsa

Day 7:

Breakfast:

- Quinoa Breakfast Bowl with Walnuts and Cinnamon

- Drink: Spiced Apple Cider with Cinnamon and Cloves

Lunch:

- Wild-Caught Salmon Salad with Arugula and Pomegranate

Snack:

- Golden Milk Energy Bites (Turmeric, Dates, and Nuts)

Dinner:

- Zucchini Noodles with Pesto and Grilled Chicken

Shopping List (for 7-Day Meal Plan)

Vegetables and Fruits:

- Kale, spinach, arugula, cucumber, zucchini, mushrooms, sweet potatoes, cauliflower, tomatoes, bell peppers, avocados, pomegranate, blueberries, bananas, pears, mango, carrots, lemons, oranges

- Fresh ginger, garlic, green onions, fresh herbs (cilantro, parsley)

Proteins:

- Wild-caught salmon, tofu, shrimp, chicken breasts, eggs, lentils, chickpeas, walnuts

Grains and Legumes:

- Quinoa, oatmeal, flaxseeds, chia seeds, spaghetti squash, brown rice, whole wheat wraps

Nuts, Seeds, and Oils:

- Almonds, walnuts, sesame seeds, coconut oil, olive oil, flaxseed crackers

Spices and Herbs:

- Turmeric, cinnamon, cloves, ground ginger, cumin, coriander, star anise, basil, oregano, thyme, sea salt, black pepper

Dairy-Free Alternatives:

- Almond milk, coconut milk, coconut yogurt

Other:

- Raw honey or maple syrup, balsamic glaze, tahini, miso paste, apple cider vinegar

Chapter 8

Lifestyle Practices to Enhance the Diet

Stress reduction techniques, importance of hydration, and mindful eating tips.

Incorporating a holistic approach to an anti-inflammatory lifestyle can significantly amplify the benefits of your diet. Alongside eating anti-inflammatory foods, managing stress, staying hydrated, and practicing mindful eating are essential elements for maintaining balance and overall health. Here's how these practices can contribute to your well-being:

Stress Reduction Techniques

Stress can be a major contributor to chronic inflammation in the body, affecting everything from immune function to digestion. By managing stress, you can help lower your body's production of pro-inflammatory hormones, particularly cortisol. Here are a few techniques to consider:

1. Deep Breathing Exercises:

Practice deep breathing techniques such as diaphragmatic breathing, where you breathe deeply through your diaphragm, not just shallowly through your chest. This helps to activate the parasympathetic nervous system, which promotes relaxation.

2.   Meditation:

Regular meditation, even for just 10-15 minutes a day, can significantly reduce stress and inflammation. Mindfulness meditation, in particular, encourages awareness of the present moment and reduces the mental stress that often exacerbates physical inflammation.

3.   Yoga and Stretching:

Yoga is known for reducing stress, improving flexibility, and calming the nervous system. Gentle poses combined with deep breathing can help lower cortisol levels and support joint and muscle health. Simple stretches throughout the day can also help release tension from the body.

4.   Progressive Muscle Relaxation (PMR):

This technique involves tensing and relaxing each muscle group in the body, one at a time. It can help reduce both physical and mental stress, promoting a sense of overall relaxation.

5.   Journaling or Expressive Writing:

Writing down your thoughts and feelings can help process emotions, relieve mental tension, and reduce stress. It's a great way to reflect on the day and release any pent-up frustrations.

Importance of Hydration

Water plays a crucial role in reducing inflammation and supporting overall health. Proper hydration helps transport nutrients, flush out toxins, and maintain the health of every cell in your body. Here's why staying hydrated is important in an anti-inflammatory diet:

1.   Flushes Out Toxins:

Water helps your kidneys filter and eliminate waste products from your body. Staying hydrated supports detoxification processes, which is vital for reducing systemic inflammation.

2. Supports Joint Health:

Hydration is essential for keeping joints lubricated, which is especially important for those experiencing inflammation in the joints, such as those with arthritis. Drinking plenty of water can help ease discomfort and improve mobility.

3. Boosts Digestion:

Proper hydration aids in digestion and prevents constipation. A healthy gut is integral to reducing inflammation and maintaining a balanced immune system. Drinking water can also prevent bloating, which may arise from inflammation.

4. Reduces Headaches and Fatigue:

Dehydration can cause headaches, dizziness, and fatigue. Staying hydrated can help prevent these symptoms and support mental clarity and physical energy levels.

5. Promotes Healthy Skin:

Hydration is key for maintaining healthy, glowing skin. Well-hydrated skin is more resilient and less prone to inflammation and conditions like eczema and psoriasis.

Hydration Tip: Aim to drink at least 8 glasses (64 oz) of water per day, but more may be needed depending on your activity level, climate, and personal needs. You can also incorporate herbal teas, coconut water, and water-rich fruits and vegetables like cucumbers and watermelon into your daily intake.

Mindful Eating Tips

Mindful eating involves paying full attention to the eating experience and appreciating the flavors, textures, and sensations of your food. It can help you develop a healthier relationship with food and prevent overeating, which can contribute to inflammation. Here are some tips for practicing mindful eating:

1.   Slow Down and Savor:

Take your time with each bite. Chew thoroughly and savor the flavors of the food. This allows your body to properly digest the food and signals to your brain when you're full, helping to avoid overeating.

2.   Eat Without Distractions:

Try to eat in a quiet environment without distractions like TV, smartphones, or computers. This allows you to focus solely on your meal, improving digestion and preventing you from eating out of stress or habit.

3.   Engage Your Senses:

Notice the colors, textures, smells, and flavors of your food. Engaging your senses helps you appreciate the experience of eating and can prevent overeating by making you more aware of when you're satisfied.

4.   Listen to Your Body:

Pay attention to your body's hunger and fullness cues. Eat when you're hungry, and stop when you're satisfied—not stuffed. Learning to tune into your body's signals can help maintain a healthy weight and support your digestive system.

5.   Practice Gratitude:

Before eating, take a moment to express gratitude for the food you have and the nutrients it provides. This practice can shift your mindset and help you approach meals with a sense of appreciation and mindfulness.

6.   Portion Control:

Mindful eating can also help you naturally practice portion control. Instead of eating large portions, take smaller bites and check in with yourself regularly to see if you're still hungry.

By incorporating these stress reduction techniques, prioritizing hydration, and practicing mindful eating, you can significantly reduce inflammation and improve your overall health. These habits complement an anti-inflammatory diet and can help you lead a healthier, more balanced life.

Made in United States
Troutdale, OR
05/19/2025